T

MW00986773

"A must-read for anybody who is interested in keeping the brain active and young. This wonderful book can be used as a practical guide for those patients looking to help themselves, as well as for healthcare providers interested in improving their patient's cognitive abilities."—*Dr. Anna Potash, psychiatrist*

"This book is written in easy to read language, especially for the aging population. Dr. Bragin introduces the brilliant innovative idea to use our developmental pathways from early childhood for activating the aging and stressed-out brain. The book is extremely valuable for physicians—like myself—who want to help their patients to optimize physical rehabilitation treatment outcomes, and for patients who want to keep the brain active."—*Dr. Mikhail Shapiro, lifetime board-certified physical and rehabilitation medicine physician, Preventive Biomedicine Center*

"This excellent and easy-to-read book provides new hope for patients and new tools for their doctors. As an osteopathic physician treating not only the physical body but also emotional impact of illnesses, I have witnessed a lot of positive results using this program. I clearly see better treatment outcome for those patients who improved their brain activity."—*Dr. Leonid Tafler, board-certified family and osteopathic physician, Osteopathic Family Health Center*

"If I were asked to characterize Dr. Bragin's book *How to Activate Your Brain* in two words, I would say: 'Optimism and Care'. From a young age, we absorbed an idea that neurons can not be revived and you can not fight the aging process. But Dr. Bragin's book gives people Hope and the Will to fight. In my opinion, this is the cornerstone of success. The book is not a theoretical textbook; it is a practical guide filled with warm and sincere care for us—the readers. It almost feels like it is not a doctor instructing his patients but a loving son giving advice to his parents. The care that the author has for the elderly can be seen even in the format and size of font, which makes the book easy to read. I just want to say 'Thank you.'"—***Ester Fayenson***

"This book is a delight to read—a splendid collection of methods and exercises that I have been using for many years. I am still functioning on a high intellectual level and do creative work despite my advanced age, only because I use these exercises on a daily basis. The exercises became my 'best friends.' I am very grateful to Dr. Bragin and the staff of his Center. I recommend this book to anyone who wants to keep their brain active for a long time." —***Samuel Gil, Ph.D.***

"This is an informative, optimistic, and accessible book for the elderly (and not so elderly) who are interested in preserving and improving their brain function. Dr. Bragin has done extensive work for creating a unique, original set of exercises and methods to help reduce stress, enhance your mind, and keep your brain active. His methods and exercises are very straightforward, and the large font makes the book very easy to read."—***Vladimir Smotkin***

How to Activate Your Brain

A Practical Guide
Book 1

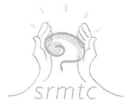

Valentin Bragin, M.D., Ph.D.

Bloomington, IN   authorHOUSE®   Milton Keynes, UK

AuthorHouse™
1663 Liberty Drive, Suite 200
Bloomington, IN 47403
www.authorhouse.com
Phone: 1-800-839-8640

AuthorHouse™ UK Ltd.
500 Avebury Boulevard
Central Milton Keynes, MK9 2BE
www.authorhouse.co.uk
Phone: 08001974150

First published by AuthorHouse 1/16/2007

ISBN: 978-1-4259-8289-8 (sc)

Library of Congress Control Number: 2006910898

Printed in the United States of America
Bloomington, Indiana

This book is printed on acid-free paper.

Cover design by E. Sedova

This book and the material in it are intended for educational purposes only.

Exercises detailed in this book must be conducted while taking into consideration the general state of the person's health.

The author makes no claim with regard to physical healing, and does not offer this book as a treatment for cognitive decline or mental disorders.

The exercises and methods in this book should NOT be used as a substitute for medical advice in diagnosing or treating any medical condition. You should consult your physician. The author and publisher disclaim any liability arising directly or indirectly from the use of this book.

Dedication

This book is dedicated to my late father and mother, Ilya and Maria Bragin.

My father was a navy doctor and a bright, talented person with an analytical mind. He instilled in me a fascination with the human body and the passion to become a doctor. He has always been my irreplaceable adviser, role model, and teacher, especially during the first years of my medical career and while I worked on my thesis. I always felt his warmth and support.

My mother was a navy nurse during WWII who later became a lawyer. She had an open heart, was a compassionate woman with deep intuition, and always believed in me and expressed her unconditional love for me. I was fortunate to spend a lot of time with her during my childhood. I was taught to do handiwork, to be a keen observer, and to control my emotions and behavior.

Contents

Acknowledgments

I will always remember comrades, teachers, and friends who contributed to my personal growth and development. The list dates back to the 1960s, when I was a medical cadet at the Medical Military Academy in Leningrad, in the former USSR.

First, I would like to thank my medical cadet group, which we called "Quintet." The group consisted of Vladimir Nebishinetz, Aleksey Zaytsev, Viktor Shindin, Victor Gnoyevoy, and me. For more than three years, we spent days and nights in the biochemistry lab, studying muscle metabolism, exchanging ideas, inspiring, helping, and supporting each other. We always believed that our shared destiny was to become good doctors and researchers. We all participated in weekly meetings—held every Thursday in the office of the head of the biochemistry department—to discuss the results of our individual projects. It was an unforgettable experience that transformed us into genuine researchers.

I wish to thank my close friend, the late Dmitry Arbisman, M.D., Ph.D., with whom I did research and had fruitful, timeless, passionate discussions about biochemical functions of different organs.

I have been fortunate to have great teachers: Professors Ilya Ilyich Ivanov, Victor Konstantinovich Kulagin, Victor Victorovich Davidov, and my biochemistry mentor and coach, Yuri Yurievich Keerig, all of whom shared their knowledge and love for research and medicine with us.

The late professor Ilya Ilyich Ivanov, head of the biochemistry department of the Medical Military Academy, taught me how to apply "chemical logic" to biochemical research. He generously shared his knowledge, experience, and research techniques, and helped me develop into a fully mature independent researcher. The late professor Victor Konstantinovich Kulagin, M.D., Ph.D., head of the pathophysiology department of the Medical Military Academy, introduced me to the concept of stress and taught me to understand various levels of physical processes that take place during the onset of stress or disease. Professor Victor Victorovich Davidov, M.D., Ph.D. worked side-by-side with me, offering constant support and encouragement during our joint projects.

The late Yuri Yurievich Keerig, M.D., Ph.D., was a "genie" for the whole group of cadets. He cultivated a deeply philosophical state of mind and was persistent and patient with research. He was our first teacher, and radiated support, encouragement, openness, caring, and warmth. He injected the love of the research into our minds.

I especially extend my most sincere thanks to my family, for this was truly a collaborative family project:

My wife Katya, for her love, patience, support, in-house editing, and helpful suggestions.

My son Ilya, who worked with me on this project doing statistical analysis, presenting our data at conferences, and making invaluable comments and suggestions.

My brother Alex, who helped me with material in the early stages of the manuscript.

My stepson David Mondrus, for his technical computer support and energetic encouragement.

Special thanks to my daughter-in-law, Marlene Mondrus, for always being available to read and edit abstracts, presentations, and articles. Her comments and corrections were of great value to me.

My love and gratitude go to my grandchildren, Nicole and Dylan. Watching them develop, grow, and learn from the world around them helped me to refine some of the exercises in this program.

My appreciation goes to my cousin, Gennady Ekht, for helping with photo and layout preparation; and to his daughter, Vera Ekht, for her comments.

There are many other people to thank for their contributions to this book:

My deep appreciation goes to the staff of the Stress Relief and Memory Training Center, who helped with the Brain Activation Program.

I would like to acknowledge each of my patients, with whom I grew as a doctor and from whom I always gained valuable feedback. I am particularly grateful to Leonid Kogan, Gavriil Levinzon, Grigory Muravin, and Dr. Leonid Berdichevsky, for their careful reading of this manuscript in Russian.

I am very grateful to Irina Slepchina, Inna Shlapko and Elena Sherbakov for their contributions to the quality of this work, valuable comments and suggestions.

Special thanks to Dr. Jon Kabat-Zinn and Saki Santorelli for the unique experience of their "Mindfulness-based Stress Reduction in Mind-Body Medicine" retreat. I found Dr. Jon Kabat-Zinn's book very useful to my practice.[1*]

Finally, many thanks to my staff member, Leonid Katsov, who assisted with graphics for this book; to freelance writer Tom Kerr, for proofreading, edits, and revisions; to freelance Russian-to-English translator Polina Skibinskaya *(www.polina-skibinskaya.com)* and to cover designer Elena Sedova *(www.rabbitteam.com)*.

*See Selected References

Dear Readers,

Your comments are always welcomed and appreciated! We have developed brain activation workshops based on this book that can be presented upon request. If you would like to share your opinion about the book or participate in these workshops, please contact me at:

Valentin Bragin, M.D., PhD.
Stress Relief and Memory Training Center
** (SRMTC)**
3101 Ocean Parkway Suite 1A
Brooklyn, NY 11235
Phone: (718) 946-2481
Website: *http://www.activateyourbrain.com*

Preface

We all know the drill. If you're sick, you need to take a rest and refrain from physical exercises. Stay in bed. Don't walk. Over and over, we are told that decreased physical activity will help our bodies fight disease. But for people who suffer from decreased concentration and memory, anxiety and depression, my advice is quite the opposite: spend less time in bed, **do more walking, and be more physically active.**

For the last twelve years, I have been working with severely ill geriatric patients at the Stress Relief and Memory Training Center, which I founded in 1994 and have headed ever since. During this work, I have developed the Brain Activation Program for elderly Russian-speaking patients suffering from a combination of serious medical and emotional problems, and decreased memory and concentration. The core of the program is a set of light physical exercises that are done mostly in a sitting position. During program development, my patients have been active collaborators, invaluable partners, and critics. They learned the program in the office and continued to use it at home.

In the process of program creation, we took into account our patients' limited physical abilities. These light physical exercises are very simple, well-tolerated, and easy to learn and remember. For several years, we handed out pamphlets for different exercises.

In 2005, in response to my patients' requests, I published *How to Activate Your Brain* in Russian.[2] We have been utilizing this book in our center ever since. The present book in English has been updated and extended.

This book consists of four parts:

Part 1 is a description of some stress-relief techniques, well-tolerated by elderly patients.

Part 2 illustrates light physical exercises that help activate brain functions, especially coordination, attention, and concentration.

Part 3 consists of a set of exercises that help strengthen memory.

Part 4 has a brief description of how food, music, and light help to activate the brain.

If the material presented in the preface and introduction of the book seems to be difficult for you, please skip these sections and go directly to the exercises.

I hope that this book will help you keep your brain healthy and happy for years to come.

Introduction

After decades of intensive research into one of the greatest mysteries on earth—the human brain—there is absolutely no doubt that the brain has an extraordinary ability to restore its own functions.

Every day, new data from numerous studies are revealed that support and confirm the existence of this important and amazing quality of the brain.

The studies are usually conducted with healthy individuals. But when they undergo stress or feel overwhelmed by mounting problems, these otherwise healthy people experience low productivity, lethargy and fatigue, shorter attention spans, and diminished memory and concentration.

But what about those people who suffer from serious medical illnesses, are chronically forgetful, inattentive, and depressed, those individuals whose brain functions become disorganized and disintegrated? These people become slower, are no longer capable of processing information quickly, and they lose their ability to make decisions. Is it possible for such people to reactivate their brain functions?

Even as recently as ten years ago, I did not have an answer to that question. The outlook was bleak and did not seem promising. For centuries, the widely accepted opinion among doctors had been that "brain cells do not regenerate." Ailing people with diminished brain functioning had little hope of ever getting better.

Today's doctors, however, understand the brain differently, and based on countless studies conducted within the past decade, and data accumulated in our own research center, we know that the brain can be activated or reactivated at virtually any age.

Significant work to improve the brain's function in an aging population is already underway all over the world. The most recent program to be developed for people of advanced age—the Nintendo Brain Age program—came to the U.S.A. from Japan in April 2006.

My staff and I have been privileged to work with elderly patients for several years. During that time, we have personally witnessed the great strides made by patients who have used these new brain activation therapies. They experienced a remarkable improvement in their brain speed (reaction time), coordination, attention, concentration, and memory. They also regained their self-confidence and optimism.

Patients find it easy to learn the various exercises offered in the program, and they have diligently practiced these exercises within our office.

The Brain Activation Program has withstood the test of time—but the work has just begun and continues to expand. With the help of my staff at the center—and the cooperation of my wonderful patients—we are constantly developing new and more advanced exercises to help stimulate and activate the brain.

My Long Path to the Brain: A Bit of History

My journey into studying about the brain functions was neither easy nor straightforward.

I came to psychiatry after twenty years of clinical and experimental practice in medicine in the former Soviet Union. During that time, I had treated various patients and worked in biochemical and pathophysiological laboratories. Besides being involved in several long-term projects, I also studied muscle protein development after birth, energy metabolism under different types of physical stresses, lung and erythrocyte metabolism, and many other related issues. But no matter which projects I did, the subject of the brain's reaction to different diseases was always on my mind.

Later, in New York, I was fortunate to work with Dr. Bill Wallace at the department of psychiatry in the Mount Sinai School of Medicine (New York). The state-of-the-art laboratory was an inspiring place. As a new immigrant, I felt like a kid in a candy store. The lab was stocked with every gadget I could possibly need, and my colleagues offered constant help and support, encouraging me to use my former research experience. In that laboratory, I studied amyloid protein synthesis in the cerebral cortex in the experimental model of Alzheimer's disease.[3,4]

Later, during my four years as a psychiatric resident, my knowledge of the human brain grew by leaps and bounds. The psychiatry of the '90s was quite different from the psychiatry I had studied at my alma mater in the '60s. It was no longer only a descriptive science. By the end of the twentieth century, psychiatry had blossomed into a science based on genetics, neurochemistry, neurophysiology, radiology, and many other disciplines.

After finishing my residency, I delved into work with patients whose medical illnesses were almost always accompanied by emotional and cognitive problems (e.g. depression, anxiety, and decreased attention and memory). Many of them were at different stages of Alzheimer's disease, which gradually eats away the brain's cognitive functions. I found that the exercises outlined in this workbook could be applied to people with different levels of cognitive deficit, from mild cognitive impairment (ambulatory patients) to the advanced stages of diseases (homebound patients). Patients and family members who were able to observe the effect of mental activation were grateful for even small positive changes.

For me, the study of the brain is a fascinating and gratifying ongoing project, especially when there is an opportunity to see the practical results of my work. I believe this is the most exciting project of my entire medical career.

My Mission

While working with chronic patients, I have witnessed different people's reactions to stress and illness. Many of the patients have strong faith in medicine only, and do not realize that they can also use the body's natural ability to heal itself along with their regular medical treatment.

It is well known that any patient has to be an active partner for successful treatment. I am always telling my patients that the treatment "starts at the office and continues at home," and that everybody has the unique set of bodily reserves that should be drawn upon on a regular basis for healing.

The mission of this book is to educate people about the brain's amazing capacity for self-repair and the possibility to activate brain function at any age, starting today.

I hope this book provides important, easy-to-digest information which can be used for many years to come.

Symptoms of an Ailing Brain

Our brain activity is constantly changing, twenty-four hours a day, during the different tasks we perform and even while we rest. If you've ever observed an electroencephalogram (EEG)—a device that records electrical signals in the brain—you've seen evidence of this firsthand.

Here are just a few factors that can impede the brain's activity:

- *Stress*
- *Aging*
- *Decrease in muscular activity and joint flexibility*
- *Extremely loud music*
- *Information overload*
- *Decrease in the oxygen supply to neurons due to problems with local blood circulation in the brain*
- *Destruction of brain cells as a result of trauma, metabolic imbalance, and other medical conditions.*

For practical purposes, based on my experience, signs of diminished brain activities include:
- *Marked diminishment of all sensory activities (e.g. vision, hearing, touch, etc.)*

- *Apparent decrease in attention and concentration*
- *Problems memorizing new information as well as recalling well known information*
- *Difficulty in making decisions*
- *Slowness and difficulty walking*
- *Problems in coordination between various parts of the body*
- *Increased number of mistakes during the execution of both simple and complex tasks*
- *Passivity, apathy, and loss of interest*

Additional problems include difficulty reading and watching television, missing important pieces of information in the news, losing the thread of conversation, repeating the same questions over and over again, and not being eager to participate in conversation at all. Often, misplacing things make people increasingly suspicious and nervous, and ultimately they accuse others of stealing. Using the stove, locking the door, and even walking, become very difficult tasks.

In a more advanced stage of brain disintegration, the person loses the ability to properly use his fingers or initiate walking and other simple actions. In my practice, there are many people who have problems performing functions requiring the simultaneous use of fingers on both hands. Their fingers become strangers, growing more and more uncontrollable, disobedient, and clumsy. In this stage, the patient's brain has probably forgotten how to repeat even the simplest movements.

What happens inside the brain to cause such drastic changes in memory and behavior?

As we age and the brain becomes diseased, many of the neurons no longer work normally, and some of them even die. The contacts between the neurons become disrupted or disappear completely. As these contacts fail, the various parts of the brain lose their ability to communicate with one another, and as a result become isolated. The disintegration proceeds gradually and spreads throughout the brain to varying degrees. The deterioration can take years before it gets to a point that a person notices something is wrong.

Gradually, they notice problems with balance and walking, focus and concentration, and memory. But in most cases, there are various brain functions and movements that remain intact and are preserved. I can always zero in on the functions and movements that have not yet been touched by disease, and then I use them to counteract the process of disintegration and activate the brain.

Birth of the Program

In 1997, I was in a three-year-old private practice and had a pretty good sense of my patients. Based on this experience, it seemed like an opportune time to look around for ways to optimize treatment protocols for our patients. As a medical doctor with more than twenty years of experience, I knew about the body's amazing restorative capacity. As a "young" psychiatrist, with seven years of experience, I had to find a treatment that would allow the fracturing, disjointed brain to work better.

Using a medical model that I had learned at my alma mater, "Treat the patient, not the illness," I started looking for literature about different types of interventions, and I attended several conferences and workshops.

Around the same time, Dr. Khalsa's book, *Brain Longevity,* arrived.[5] The information within this book was very helpful for me and it strengthened my thoughts about the real possibility of treating the aging brain from different angles.

I attended the yearly Traumatic Brain Injury Conference in Williamsburg that same year, and found the experience very inspirational for our work.

In the beginning, there were many more questions than answers. How can we help an aging brain that is already at a level of disintegration and disengagement? How can we evaluate the extent of disintegration, and determine what reserve capacity still remains in the brain? What kinds of exercises are safe for patients with severe medical conditions?

By that time, I already had the basic elements of the program in mind. They included strategies for combating stress, dietary recommendations, physical exercise, attention and memory training, medications, vitamins, music and light stimulation.

Physical exercise had to be the cornerstone of the program. As far as the design of the types of physical exercises within the program, and their magnitude, I did not yet have a clear idea. But I did list a set of requirements for physical exercises for severely ill patients. The criteria that I established for the exercises were as follows:

- *Very easy to comprehend and implement*
- *Done mostly while seated*
- *Gradually extending from single to multiple muscle groups*
- *Consisting of different intensities and frequencies*
- *Individually tailored to each patient*

Our goal was to preserve cognitive function in elderly patients by any means, for as long as possible.

As the cache of exercises grew between 1997 and 2002, research was also growing. Published studies repeatedly proved that we were on the right track: The brain could, and did, access its reserves to fight the disease.

To illustrate the process by which the exercises in the program were created, I'd like to talk about my experience with two particular patients.

Patient M.

While M. was in the advanced stages of Alzheimer's disease, he was brought to the office by his wife. He had long ago stopped recognizing his loved ones, and had lost almost all of his ability to speak.

I picked up a thick, round, walking stick and put it into M's hands. He clutched the stick firmly with both hands. I began rotating the stick slowly and M. followed my lead and rotated the stick along with me.

We silently spent five minutes on this exercise. At the end of the session, M. turned to his wife and, clearly and with confidence, said the word "woman."

M.'s wife was amazed. It had been several months since he'd spoken clearly. Based on this breakthrough with M., I created **Exercise 4.8, Pencil**.

Patient D.

D. came to me with moderate attention and memory decline. For example, he could not perform the simple physical activity of balling one hand into a fist while simultaneously unclenching the other hand.

We gave D. a tennis ball and asked him to try again. He clenched and unclenched his hands flawlessly, creating **Exercise 4.9, Tennis Ball**.

Recently, we collected data showing that the **Tennis Ball** exercise can also have a beneficial effect on the heart rate variability (HRV). The results of this observation were presented at the International Conference on Prevention of Dementia in Washington in 2005.[6]

Various parts of the exercises were well-received by the vast majority of patients who agreed to participate in the program. Physical exercises also decreased the anxiety of many patients and improved their mood. One of my patients noted, "When I'm doing the exercises, no thoughts enter into my mind. I feel much better after exercises."

Program Description

Figure 1 shows the essential elements of the Brain Activation Program:

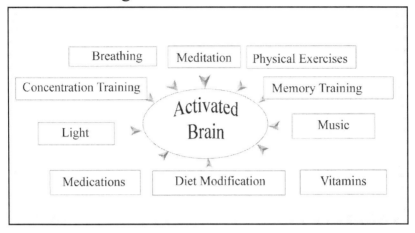

Figure 1 Brain Activation Program

The Brain Activation Program consists of:

1. The development of a positive mindset and reasonable expectations for working with the program.
2. Breathing and meditation done separately as well as simultaneously.
3. Light physical exercises for various muscle groups.
4. Concentration, attention, and coordination training during physical exercise.
5. Training for different types of memory (of objects, pictures, shapes, etc.). Both medical

and popular literature describe countless techniques and regimens which help strengthen memory.[7,8,9,10] In this book, we will talk specifically about a few practical ways for elderly people to strengthen memory.

6. Exposure to light and music for relaxation as well as stimulation of the brain.

7. Activating the brain's metabolic activity through a regular regimen of medications, vitamins, minerals, and nutritional supplements.

As I mentioned before, sets of physical exercises are the key elements in this program. They were developed in the office through many hours of working with patients who had varying mental capacities for processing and repeating movements. During the period of development and selection of exercises, we were constantly doing an analysis of the patient's ability to learn and tolerate the exercises and to do homework. Our goal in this part of the program was to achieve the maximum effect on brain activation and concentration with minimal physical exertion.

From research and literature on the subject, we know that every movement activates a certain number of brain cells and the connections between them. The longer we exercise, the more active contacts are created—and the stronger the existing ones become. The memory of long-forgotten movements returns to us, and flexibility of small joints is restored. Brain functions then become more active and synchronized.

Theory Behind the Program

Every day brings us new knowledge about the brain's functions. To better understand the way this exercise program works, I would like to introduce a few facts about the development of the body, especially regarding the connections between the brain and muscles.

First theoretical suggestion:

Muscular activity has a profound effect on the development and function of our nervous system. Communications go back and forth between the brain and muscles all the time. This begins even before birth, and after birth there are major increases in the brain and muscle communications.

In the '60s, our group was studying contraction protein accumulation in the heart and muscles of newborn rabbits.[11] In the heart, there was a slow accumulation of these contraction proteins, which are special proteins that aid in the flexing of muscle fiber. In the muscles, we found a drastic increase of the same proteins by the end of two weeks after birth, when an animal stopped crawling and started jumping.

One of the possible explanations for this increase was based on different protein functions in the heart and muscles. The heart started working much earlier, in the womb, and did not show major transformations after birth. But muscles did not fully develop in the embryo stage. After birth, however, muscles became active with increased protein synthesis and amazing changes in movement, from crawling all the way to jumping.

In humans, the transition from crawling to walking to running takes several months. This is a special time for babies, during which the maturation of brain communications between the brain and muscles help to produce movements. But for other newborn mammals (e.g. cats, dogs, and primates), this time period is much shorter than it is for humans. Newborn horses and cows can stand firmly on all four legs immediately after birth. The different timeframe of various body part development has a profound effect on nervous system maturation.

When a baby starts to crawl and stands up, these are important signs of brain development, coordination, and muscle strength. If the baby is not able to crawl or stand up on time, it means that something is going wrong with the development of the baby's nervous system. A growing baby constantly uses all the senses (sight, hearing, taste, touch, and smell), repeatedly playing with objects, touching them, and trying to put them into the mouth. This sensory stimulation and muscle movements activate the brain and help it grow and develop.

I was recently observing my baby grandson as he desperately tried to turn over while lying on his back. The baby repeated the same movements hundreds of times with amazing persistence. Finally, the baby succeeded and turned over. But he felt no sense of triumph after all his efforts. He did not take a break. Instead, the child kept turning over until he learned to do it quickly and easily.

Observing his self-training, I thought that first of all, he probably enjoyed the process of movement. And secondly, he gathered together his attention and concentration to accomplish the task. The key to the child's success was his constant repetition of the movements, an unwavering desire to perfect the task, a deep level of concentration, and strength of will and determination. Within a few months, he started to stand up, and when learning to stand, he performed this action multiple (more than 100) times. He was not tired. He simply enjoyed the process.

While pondering his training process, it became very clear to me that our brain is probably genetically programmed to do multiple repetitions while learning any kind of movement. The more repetitions you perform, the better it is for the brain. For noticeable and measurable training results, the number of repetitions has to exceed 100.

Second theoretical suggestion:

It is a well-known fact that in the adult brain, the sensory-motor zone of the cerebral cortex is not evenly split between control of different body parts.

That means that the strength of the connections between the brain's cerebral cortex and the various parts of the body are not always the same. They differ depending on which part of the body is connected to the cerebral cortex of the brain. This fact is probably a result of how we develop in the early stages of life.

The parts of the body that develop sooner and are the most active are the parts that correspond with the largest areas in the brain. In other words, the sooner we use a part of our body, and the more we use it, the more area in the brain is devoted to connecting with that part of the body.

In the early months of a baby's life, the parts of the body we call "mimic muscles"—which include the muscles that control the face, the tongue, the larynx, and the hands—are most often used. As result, those parts of the body occupy the largest portion of the sensory motor zone. They are given more space in the cerebral cortex of the brain, because of how important they are when babies begin to develop.

Children in the first twelve months use their hands more actively than their legs. And in the adult brain, the area corresponding to the hands is much larger than the brain area that corresponds to the legs.

What happens to the brain as we grow older?

It seems that those parts of the body that become active earlier in our development stay active longer in life, and vice versa. The functioning of the legs fully develops nine to ten months later than the functioning of the hands. And gait problems—the problems with keeping our balance and walking—are usually the first to emerge when we grow older. Recent studies have shown that gait problems might be an early sign of dementia.

Third theoretical suggestion:

The brain has an enormous capacity for self-repair. It has been seen for many years in the recoveries of stroke and head trauma victims. Brain plasticity is demonstrated in numerous studies.[12, 13]

Fourth theoretical suggestion:

Stress has a strong influence on brain functions, and affects the entire body, from the brain all the way to the single cell. It throws the brain out of synch, and the connections between different parts of the brain become temporarily disabled. Stress decreases concentration, focus, and memory, and causes anxiety, fear, and depression. Fighting stress is an absolutely necessary step on the way to help the brain's recovery.

Train the Brain (and Muscles, too)

The brain and muscle exercises have a lot in common: They both require determination and a full understanding of the workout's importance. For both types of training, the person has to be motivated and have a positive emotional attitude.

Physical training activates the brain, increases blood flow to the muscles and brain, and creates new muscle proteins and new neuron connections. Physical exercise requires a great deal of attention, coordination, and the ability to remember movements. Light, simple physical exercises are easy to remember and focus on. But for more advanced physical training, our memory, attention, and concentration have to be in good shape.

Professional athletes have to maintain intense concentration for the entire length of their performance, remembering not just every movement but also the proper sequence and timing of those movements. In order to master a routine, they must practice and repeat it hundreds—and sometimes thousands—of times.

The brain's capacity to concentrate on a specific muscle group and to memorize a sequence of movements is extremely important for successful training. As we train, we learn to be aware of the position of each of our muscle groups at any given moment. It's no wonder then that when we put our muscles through a sequence of physical exercises, we are also automatically and subconsciously training our brain.

From my experience, a brain workout involves a broader concept of exercise than do ordinary physical workouts. It consists of such elements as:

- *Muscle movements, which may (or may not) be part of a physical training routine.*
- *Activation of all sensory channels (e.g. vision, hearing, touch, etc.).*

- Training of attention, concentration, and memory, by using both computerized and non-computerized techniques.

The simultaneous training of movement, concentration, and memory is a real challenge for the brain at any age. Learning to drive is a great example of this kind of simultaneous training. If you want to learn how to drive, you definitely have to learn a host of different skills. First, you must study the rules (a theoretical learning process). Then, you can move on to learning the physical skills of driving, such as steering and checking your mirrors. During this training, you always have to concentrate and remember the rules you learned. This way, you can synchronize new movements and perform many types of training all at the same time.

At first, you might have trouble achieving this synchronization or multitasking ability, and this might frustrate you. The car keeps moving in the wrong direction instead of going straight. But as you repeat the process, over and over again, your movements slowly become less awkward. You feel a growing sense of satisfaction. But this is only the beginning of your learning process.

Your next goal is to achieve a level of driving that happens automatically. Over time, it becomes second nature, and you begin controlling the car with ease, without consciously thinking about it, and you begin to truly enjoy the act of driving.

Our exercises activate the brain in the same way, starting from simple movements (and frustration), to mastering them, and then moving on to a level of performing them automatically with pleasure.

You must begin by memorizing exercises and their sequence (the order in which they are done). During this initial period of time, your head will probably fill up with lots of doubt and questions. The workout may seem too difficult to remember. But gradually, you will master the technique of the exercises, and your sense of satisfaction and accomplishment will grow. You will begin to notice improvements. Finally, there will be a moment when you begin to *enjoy* the workout process.

Another important part of brain activation and training has to be mentioned here. When you concentrate on the exercises, your brain no longer has time and energy to worry about other things. The exercises chase away anxiety and depression, and your emotional well-being improves. Just by memorizing and doing the exercises, you will feel successful and be filled with pride and a sense of empowerment.

How Physical Activity Influences the Brain

Let's take a brief and closer look at the way physical activity influences the brain. Physical exercise:

- *Activates the brain, no matter how old we are*
- *Increases the flow of blood, oxygen, and glucose to the different parts of the brain*
- *Triggers intensive production of different "signal" molecules (peptides) in the brain. These chemicals activate the network of new contacts (synapses) between the cells in the brain[14]*
- *Requires concentration and attention, which are important factors in memory, since the process of memory begins with concentration*
- *Is a natural way to activate the brain starting from early childhood*
- *Takes attention away from worry, anxiety, and even depression.*

Our Experience with the Program

As the Brain Activation Program was implemented at the Stress Relief and Memory Training Center, we constantly improved the exercises contained in the program, based on patients' feedback.

In the beginning, the patients came to us complaining of:

- *lack of attention*
- *forgetfulness*
- *feeling depressed and apathetic*
- *experiencing anxiety and worry*

Based on objective measures, we found that most of our patients experienced deficiency in sensory-motor coordination between the fingers, hands, and legs, and had problems with attention, concentration, and memory. Some of the patients (roughly 25 percent) who complained of forgetfulness had also experienced problems with concentration and attention.

Based on these data, we offered brain activation programs that were individually designed to suit the needs of each patient. After six months of treatment, there was a marked improvement in brain speed (reaction time), coordination, attention, concentration, and memory.

These improvements showed no signs of receding, up to twenty-four months into the program. Results of these observations were presented at several medical conferences held between the years 2000 and 2005. In 2005, the findings were featured in a scientific journal.[15]

Before you begin the Brain Activation Program, ask yourself these questions:

- What is my goal?
- What do I hope to achieve?

Setting Personal Goals

By reading this book, you took the first step on the road to activating your brain. I hope this book becomes your constant companion and will help to reach your goals. Before you can reach them, however, you must decide what they are. Filling in the information form below will help you plan your work.

What are your goals with this program?

1. _____

2. _____

3. _____

4. _____

5. _____

What results do you hope to achieve?

1. _____

2. _____

3. _____

4. _____

5. _____

How to Use This Book

To work successfully with this program, you need:

✓ Pen (or pencil) and paper
✓ Clock (with a second hand)
✓ Tennis ball
✓ Bottle of water

The first step is to read this book and learn the exercises, within two to three weeks.

The second step is to develop your personal strategy for implementing these exercises. It is very important to use a clock while performing the exercises. From my experience working with the program, the brain has to be engaged during twelve to fifteen minutes of exercise, two or more times a day. In all types of training, the breathing and meditation (relaxation) exercises from Part 1 also have to be used.

The third step is to improve muscle coordination, attention, and concentration for three or four months. This is the most important timeframe in the Brain Activation Program.

The fourth step is to train your memory.

Along with this work, you also have to make an effort to change your eating habits, and to use music and exposure to light more actively. Medication, vitamins, and supplements should be taken only after consultation with your doctor.

How to Do the Exercises

The positive expectations and feeling of self-discovery that come as you do the exercises will make your work more interesting and effective. Motivation, perseverance, patience, and time are crucial for your success.

Start and end each day with these words:

- *My brain is working more and more effectively.*
- *My attention and concentration are getting stronger and stronger.*
- *My memory is getting better and better.*
- *My movements are getting smoother.*
- *My coordination is getting better.*

Remember: A positive attitude, breathing, meditation (relaxation), physical exercise, and concentration and memory exercises will help improve your brain functions for many years to come.

There are several simple and practical rules before you start exercising:
1. Eliminate all distractions (turn off the TV, radio, phone, etc.).
2. Find a clock that shows seconds.
3. Do the exercises only in a sitting position.
4. Do the exercises at the same time every day.
5. Repeat the exercise regimen several times a day.
6. Do not skip days.
7. Do not push yourself beyond your limits.

During the workout, notice how long it takes for you to feel the first signs of exhaustion, and then stop exercising. This is your threshold for the day. Write down the length of your workout and your feelings during the exercises in your exercise diary. Over time, you will find that more stamina and endurance will be developed.

Decrease Day-to-Day Anxiety

It is very important to eliminate possible sources of everyday worries, anxiety, and fears that you frequently encounter. These are slowly destroying your brain. Examples of things that stress and worry you could include: misplacing important papers, documents, photos, money, and keys. Forgetting to turn off ovens and stoves, leaving lights on, and forgetting to close and lock doors are also powerful sources of fear and worry.

When you have to find something and don't remember where you put it, don't panic. With time, you will recall where it is. Try to replay in your mind when you last saw it. Try to remember what else was happening at that time. Stay calm and you will find it much sooner than you would if you panic.

To help you free yourself of unnecessary negative emotions:

- *Try to reserve special places for important items and keep them only in these locations.*

- Write down in a notebook where you keep all your important things and documents. Make several copies of this information and give them to your closest relative or a person you trust.
- Develop a habit of repeating your actions in the future, present, and past tense. Then, you'll be sure to remember!

For example, if you have to remember to turn off the stove, repeat:

- I will turn off the stove.
- I am turning off the stove.
- I turned off the stove.

Or if you have to remember to lock the front door, repeat:

- I will lock the top (or bottom) lock.
- I am locking the top (or bottom) lock.
- I locked the top (or bottom) lock.

Now you are ready to begin the Brain Activation Program.
Good luck in your adventure!

Dr. Valentin Bragin

Part I:
Fighting the Stress

What Happens to Our Bodies under Stress?

Ever since the Canadian scientist Hans Selye discovered stress, studies of stress have continued to capture our attention, especially in the contemporary world, where people are regularly exposed to traumatic events. "Stress" is one of the most widely used terms in today's society. The number of publications regarding stress is still on the rise, and this information has moved from academic medical journals to mainstream pop culture magazines.

Stress is a process which ignites in the body under the influence of stress factors and continues for a period of time. When stress occurs, a cascade of information is relayed from the sensory systems to the brain and then back down to hormonal systems, organs, and even to single cells in the body. Under stress, an organism quickly moves to a "stress state," and the intensity of the change depends on the type and strength of the stress-factor, individual sensitivity, and post-traumatic memory.

There are both acute and chronic types of stress. Acute stress is often accompanied by sudden trauma or disease. Chronic stress develops in the body in response to ongoing diseases. People of advanced age are especially vulnerable to chronic stress because of the extended nature of their illnesses and the gradual weakening of bodily functions.

There are a number of very good techniques for overcoming chronic stress; among them: relaxation techniques (progressive muscle relaxation and autogenic training biofeedback), breathing exercises, and meditation. Unfortunately, many relaxation techniques are difficult for people to perform, due to the concentration and focused attention that is required. And although many relaxation techniques prove to be difficult tasks for elderly people, breathing and simple meditation exercises have shown to be easily implemented, well tolerated, and useful for the elderly.

1. Breathing

Breathing exercises should always be used when it is time to relax your body and create a sense of well-being.

As we go about our daily business, most of us never give breathing a second thought, as it constantly fluctuates to adjust to whatever type of activity we do. For example, when we become lost in some sort of enthralling activity, we often unconsciously hold our breath. But breathing doesn't have to remain an unconscious activity; each of us can regulate it. We can switch our attention to our breathing at any time and get immediate benefit from it.

There are many types of breathing, but we will discuss only two kinds of breathing patterns (Figure

2): healthy, effective breathing ("the trapezoid pattern"); and shallow, ineffective breathing ("the saw pattern"). Healthy breathing is punctuated by short pauses. These pauses are crucial for the correct exchange of oxygen and carbon dioxide.

The Trapezoid   The Saw

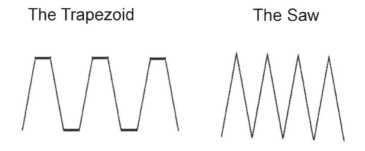

Healthy, effective breathing.   Shallow, ineffective breathing

Figure 2: Breathing Diagrams

Breathing performs another important bodily function, particularly in the lungs. Of course, everybody knows that the lungs are responsible for air exchange: They deliver oxygen to the blood and remove carbon dioxide from the blood. But few people know that the lungs are also active metabolic organs that normalize chemical compounds in the blood, which then flow to vital organs, including the heart and the brain. When the lungs receive blood with high concentrations of certain substances, the amount of those substances that goes to the heart and brain, decreases. This also works in the opposite way: When the blood, which flows to the lungs, doesn't have enough of these substances, the lungs supply them out from their own "reserves," in order to enrich the blood that reaches the heart and the brain. That is why breathing exercises and lung functions are so important—not only for the process of air exchange, but also for the essential make-up of the blood, which feeds our most vital organs, the heart and brain.

Now it is time to start the exercises. These exercises must be done in a sitting position, with your eyes closed and with full awareness of the breathing process at all times.

Exercise 1.1. Check Your Breathing.

Place your right palm on the chest area and your left palm on your abdomen or belly. Close your eyes. Breathe calmly and normally through the nose, with your usual rhythm.

If you are mostly using the upper portion of your lungs, you will notice that your right hand rises more than your left hand.

If you are using more of the middle and lower portion of your lungs, you will feel how your left hand rises and falls with each breath.

A mixed type of breathing will cause both of your hands to rise.

The following exercises will help you to activate an abdominal breathing, which is deeper and healthier. Each breathing cycle will start on inhalation or exhalation. You should patiently breathe all the way through, until a new cycle begins.

Exercise 1.2. Deep Breathing (Version 1)

In this exercise, you will start your cycle on the inhalation.

First, place your hands on the abdominal area and maintain a normal breathing rhythm for several seconds.

Now, imagine that there is a rubber ball inside your abdomen.

Inhale and notice how the abdomen swells and pushes out, and the "imaginary rubber ball" expands with air. As you exhale, pay attention to the way your stomach goes back in, as the imaginary rubber ball deflates and shrinks.

To increase the effect of this exercise, please close your eyes and be fully aware of your abdominal movements as you breathe.

Continue to breathe in this manner for several minutes, paying close attention to the inhalations and exhalations, and the expanding and retracting of your abdomen.

Exercise 1.3. Abdominal Breathing (Version 2)

In this exercise, your breathing cycle starts on exhalation.

First, place your hands on the abdominal area and maintain your regular breathing rhythm for several seconds.

Now imagine a candle burning in front of you. As you exhale, imagine blowing out the candle while you bring in your stomach. After exhaling all your air, inhale and bring your attention back, imagining that you have a lit candle in front of you, so that you can pretend to blow it out when you exhale again.

To increase an effect of this exercise, please close your eyes and concentrate on your breathing. Maintain this rhythm for several minutes, repeating the in-and-out breathing pattern.

Exercise 1.4. Abdominal Breathing (Version 3)

In this exercise, your breathing cycle starts on inhalation.

First, place your hands on the abdomen and maintain your regular rhythm for several seconds. Then, wrap your arms around your chest, as if you are giving yourself a hug.

Focus your attention on your abdomen. Inhale and notice how your abdomen extends and goes forward. As you exhale, pay attention to the way your stomach retracts. Continue breathing in this way for several minutes.

Exercise 1.5. Concentration on the Fingers

First, place your hands on your knees, with the palms open and facing up, so that the backs of your hands rest on your knees.

Then, as you inhale, bring the hands together, and touch the fingertips of one hand against the fingertips of the other hand. Pay attention as the tips of your fingers come together from each hand. Focus your full attention on the moment that the fingers touch each other. Now let your breath out, and as you exhale, move your fingers apart.

As you inhale, again, bring your thumb and your index finger together (photo 1.5.1). As you exhale, slowly move them apart.

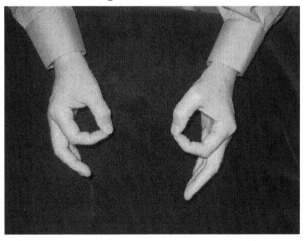

PHOTO 1.5.1.

The next time you inhale, bring your thumb and your middle finger together (photo 1.5.2). As you exhale, move them apart.

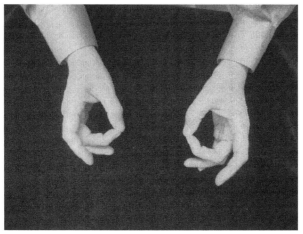

PHOTO 1.5.2.

Now, as you inhale, bring your thumb and your ring finger together (photo 1.5.3). As you exhale, move them apart.

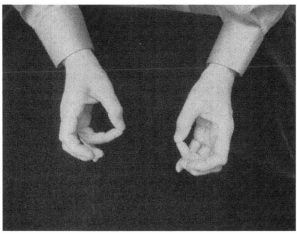

PHOTO 1.5.3.

Now, as you inhale, bring your thumb and your pinkie finger together (photo 1.5.4). As you exhale, move them apart.

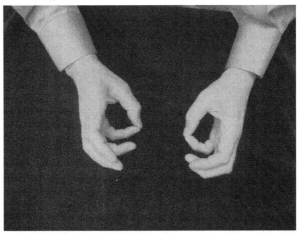

PHOTO 1.5.4.

Now, as you inhale, bring your thumb and both your index and middle fingers together (photo 1.5.5). As you exhale, move them apart.

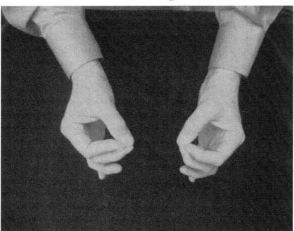

PHOTO 1.5.5.

Now, as you inhale, bring your thumb and both your ring and pinkie fingers together (photo 1.5.6). As you exhale, move them apart.

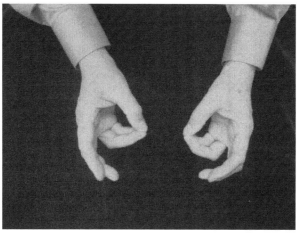

PHOTO **1.5.6.**

Now, as you inhale, bring your thumb and your index, middle, and ring fingers together (photo 1.5.7). As you exhale, move them apart.

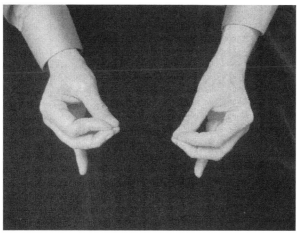

PHOTO **1.5.7.**

And finally, as you inhale, bring your thumb and your index, middle, ring, and pinkie fingers all together (photo 1.5.8). As you exhale, move them apart.

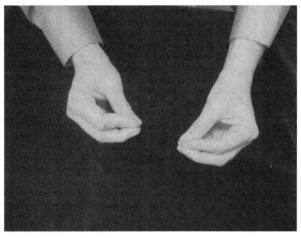

PHOTO **1.5.8.**

Exercise 1.6. Concentration on the Tennis Ball

During this exercise, your attention will be on your hands, especially at the moment when your fingers touch the ball at the end of the inhalation.

Place the tennis ball in the open palm of your right hand (photo 1.6.1).

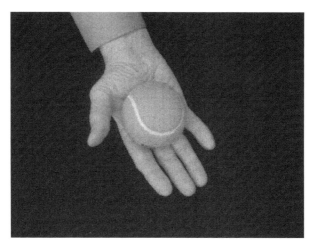

PHOTO 1.6.1.

As you inhale, wrap your fingers around the ball (photo 1.6.2).

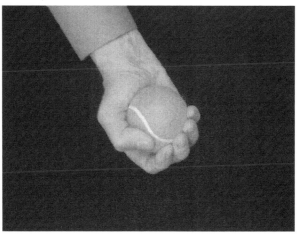

PHOTO 1.6.2.

As you exhale, open your palm again (photo 1.6.1. above).

Repeat this exercise five to ten times. Then, do the same exercise using the tennis ball in your left hand.

Next, place the ball between your palms (photo 1.6.3).

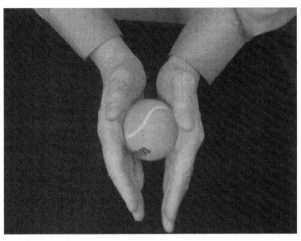

PHOTO 1.6.3.

As you inhale, let the fingers of both hands touch the ball (photo 1.6.4).

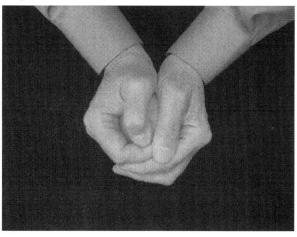

PHOTO 1.6.4.

As you exhale, open the palms of your hands (photo 1.6.3. on previous page).

Exercise 1.7. Concentration on Drinking Water

Fill a glass with clean, room-temperature drinking water. You will drink the water slowly, with small, measured sips, concentrating on your body's internal organs and systems.

In your mind, to yourself, you will say the name of an internal organ before taking each sip. Concentrate on that organ and its location in the body.

Repeat silently: **"I am concentrating on [the name of the organ] and wish it good health. I love and respect [the name of the organ]. I dedicate**

Valentin Bragin, M.D.

this sip of water to improve the well-being of [the name of the organ]."

For example:

If the organ you want to focus on is the heart, you will fill in the blank with the name of the organ "heart" as you say the phrase to yourself silently in your mind. It would be done like this:

"I am concentrating on my heart and wish it good health. I love and respect the heart. I dedicate this sip of water to improve the well-being of the heart."

In that way, dedicate the first sip to your brain, then the next sip to the heart, then a sip for the lungs, one for the liver, another sip for the gallbladder, one for the spleen, and finally take a sip for the pancreas. Continue the exercise, dedicating each slow sip to the other organs and parts of the body, including the kidneys, the bladder, the muscles, the bones, the spine, the arteries, the veins, the immune system, and so on.

End the exercise by addressing all the cells and organs in your body.

It will take approximately ten or fifteen minutes to complete this exercise.

2. Meditation

Meditation is a time-tested technique that has been used for thousands of years by people from Eastern cultures to strengthen mental and physical health. Meditation—which is a method for deep relaxation—is an indispensable brain-activation and stress-relief technique that aims at a special state of mind.

You don't have to travel to the distant and exotic Buddhist temples or Tibetan monasteries to learn the secrets of meditation. And you do not have to believe in Eastern philosophy or religion to do the meditation exercises in this book, which are not based on any religious ideas but rather on medical research. This scientific research shows how deep relaxation can help you to maintain your health and stimulate the functions of the brain.

You can use meditation at any time—as long as you can escape from distractions such as the phone, the television, the radio, or your favorite cat or dog that wants all of your attention.

For successful meditation, I recommend that you:

- *Wear light, loose-fitting clothes which will not impede your movement.*
- *Set aside a specific time when nothing will distract you.*

- *Find a quiet, comfortable spot where you won't be interrupted.*
- *Make sure the room is well-ventilated, with good clean air to breathe.*

Meditation positively affects our brain by strengthening our concentration, focus, and attention.

Simply do the following exercises and you will immediately see how helpful meditation can be!

Exercise 2.1. Sitting Meditation

Sit in a comfortable position. Put your hands on your knees with your palms facing up. Now bring the thumb and index finger of each hand together to form a small circle. Open your mouth slightly. The tip of your tongue should slightly touch the roof of your mouth, right behind your upper front teeth.

Imagine lines that connect the thumbs and index fingers of each hand and the tip of your tongue. Imagine that these lines are going from your fingertips to your tongue to form a triangle. The base of the imaginary triangle is across your knees—between your hands—and the top point of the triangle is at your tongue where it touches the roof of your mouth.

Now close your eyes and concentrate on your breathing. You might want to focus your attention on the tip of your nose, on your chest, or on your abdomen, or on any other part of your body that you want to that helps you pay attention to your breathing.

In your head, to yourself, say the words: **"Thoughts come into my mind and then they leave."**

Each time a thought enters your conscious mind, or whenever you begin to feel drowsy, simply bring your attention back to your breathing and repeat the phrase again: **"Thoughts come into my mind and then they leave."**

If you feel sleepy when the meditation is over, stretch out your arms a few times (photo 2.1).

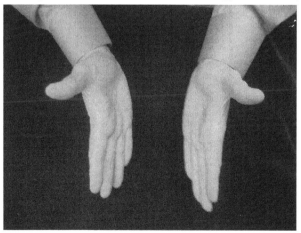

PHOTO **2.1.**

Exercise 2.2. Walking Meditation (Version 1)

Go for a walk. Walk slowly with a calm, measured pace. Place your full attention on your breathing. Try to synchronize or coordinate your movements with your breaths. For example, take two steps as you inhale, then two to four steps as you exhale. Pay attention to the sensations inside your body and your emotional state of mind. Note how they change over the course of your walk. Keep trying to pace your breathing, so that you count your steps (1, 2, 3) on the inhalation, and then count your steps (1, 2, 3) on the exhalation. Try to coordinate walking and breathing as you focus on calm stepping and breathing.

Exercise 2.3. Walking Meditation (Version 2)

Go for a walk. Walk slowly, in a calm, measured rhythm. Breathe calmly. Place your full attention on the surroundings, especially on nature. Select objects around you (for example, trees, grass, flowers, or the ocean) as a way to focus during your meditation. While walking, study the details of these objects. Observe their behavior, sounds, and movement. It might be the leaves rustling in the wind, the rays of the sun casting shadows or lighting up the grass, or the waves crashing at the shore.

Exercise 2.4. Walking Meditation (Version 3)

Go for a walk. Walk in a calm, measured pace. Place your full attention on your pace and on the sensation of your body.

At the beginning of the first step, and while you're standing still, notice how your body's weight is equally distributed and balanced between both legs. Then think about the moment when you will make the first step with your right leg. To do this, simply shift your body weight to the left leg. Raise your right foot, start the first step, and touch the ground with your right foot in front of you.

Notice how the weight shifts from the left to the right leg, and pay attention to the moment when the weight is again equally distributed between both legs. Then, put all your weight on your right leg, lift your left leg, and bring it next to the right leg. Your weight is once again distributed equally between both legs.

The next step will start with your left foot, with the same elements of movement.

Walk several minutes in this manner, and gradually increase the length of this exercise to fifteen to twenty minutes.

Part II:
Light Physical Exercises

Sets of light physical exercise involving different parts of the body (the face, hands, feet, and the spine) will be presented in this part of the book, as well as exercises which combine several parts of the body. These exercises are designed to be performed in a sitting position only. Your breathing has to be calm and even. The duration of these exercises will be controlled either by counting the number of repetitions or by keeping track of time with a clock.

Hand and face exercises are especially important. Although your face and your hands take up little space in your body, they occupy a larger part of the sensory-motor zone inside your brain than other body parts. An explanation of this phenomenon was provided in the introduction section of this book.

If you notice any unpleasant feeling while exercising, immediately stop and observe your reaction.

3. The Face, the Ears, and the Eyes

Exercise 3.1. The Face

The facial muscles, lips, and tongue play a crucial role in brain activation. You will begin your day nicely if you start it with some simple facial exercises.

Start these exercises by gently focusing your attention on the face.

1. Tense up your forehead, then relax it.
2. Squeeze your eyes shut, and then open them.
3. Keeping your teeth firmly together, open your lips as wide as you can, and then close them.
4. Keeping your lips firmly together, inflate your cheeks, and then slowly let the air out.
5. Pucker your lips, pull them in, and then move them in clockwise and counterclockwise directions several times.
6. Keeping your mouth closed, start moving your tongue inside your mouth in clockwise and counterclockwise directions. Do this several times.

Exercise 3.2. The Ears

A light ear massage activates the areas of the brain that control our hearing ability, and also has a calming effect. Touch each of your ears with your thumbs and index fingers. Focus your attention on the fingertips as they touch your ears. Take several breaths.

Rub your earlobes lightly. Move your fingertips slowly up and down, slightly massaging the front and back of the ears. For a few seconds, hold the earlobes with your thumbs and index fingers.

Valentin Bragin, M.D.

With your palms, slightly and lightly press your ears to your head. Stay in this position until you feel pleasant warmth spreading from your hands to your ears.

Exercise 3.3. The Eyes

Eye exercises activate those brain zones that are responsible for vision, as well as the strength and coordination of the eye muscles. You can use these exercises as a warm-up before any kind of training, or as a relief of fatigue.

3.3.1. Bat your eyes. Move your eyes up and down, left and right, and then roll your eyes in circles (repeat five to ten times).

3.3.2. Place your palm seven to twelve inches away from your face (in close proximity). Look at your palm, and then move your eyes to the furthest corner of the room (repeat five to ten times).

3.3.3. Gently massage the area around your eyes. Massage the skin above the eyebrows, and the outer corners of the eyes.

3.3.4. Move your eyes horizontally while simultaneously tapping the back of your left hand with the middle finger of your right hand, then change hands.

3.3.5. Repeat exercise **3.3.4,** but only move your eyes up and down, or in other words move them vertically instead of horizontally.

3.3.6. Stars. Using Figures 3 and 4, you will select one type of star to concentrate on. Touch with your right index finger the rest of the stars that have the same shape. Touch them one by one. Repeat this exercise with the other stars (the stars of other shapes).

3.3.7. Numbers. In Figures 5, 6, 7, and 8, you will find a sequence of numbers which are not in the right order; they will be all mixed up. You will have to find the numbers one at a time, in order, starting with 1, then looking for 2, then finding 3, and so forth, until you find them all.

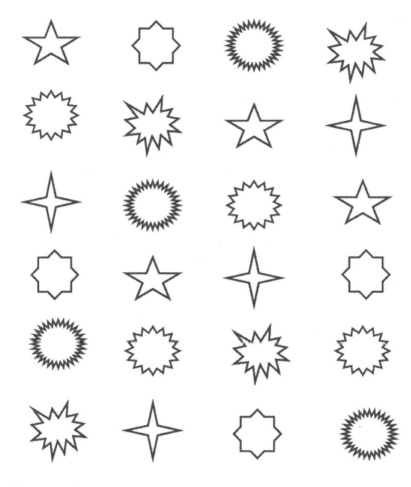

FIGURE 3

28

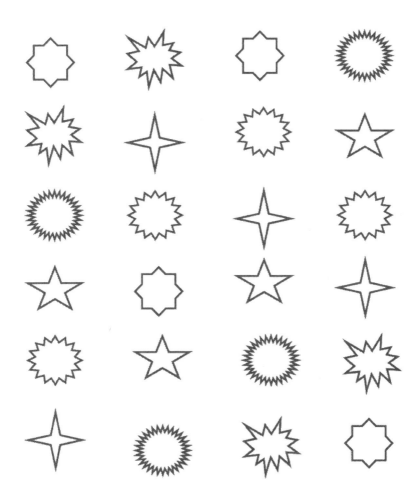

FIGURE 4

6	24	3	28
15	1	7	26
9	10	23	13
12	14	5	20
17	27	19	16
21	22	11	2
25	8	18	4

FIGURE 5

12	20	18	25
26	22	7	2
9	15	28	23
13	5	3	16
17	27	19	10
21	6	1	24
4	14	8	11

FIGURE 6

♠	9	♣	19	24
5	18	22	7	♦
♦	13	10	♣	12
25	3	♥	20	♠
♣	17	♣	15	2
21	6	♠	1	♥
23	♠	16	8	♦
♥	4	14	♥	11

FIGURE 7

16	♦	22	♥	1
7	18	♣	5	12
♣	13	15	♣	24
3	25	♥	20	♣
♣	19	2	♣	17
9	6	♦	21	♥
11	♠	10	8	♦
♥	4	1	♥	23

FIGURE 8

3.3.8. Rub your palms together until you feel pleasant warmth. Cup your palms and place them over the eye area, leaving approximately an inch of space between the palms and the eyes. Your wrists should be touching your cheekbones, and your fingers touching your forehead. Close your eyes. Focus on the pleasant warmth radiating from your palms. Open your eyes and remove your hands.

4. Hands

"Idle Hands Are the Devil's Workshop"

No matter what kind of jobs you may have done over the years, you have spent your entire lifetime using your hands. But as we grow older, we begin to notice that moving our fingers and holding things in our hands becomes increasingly awkward. We sometimes fumble or drop things, and may begin to lose confidence in our dextcrity.

What is going on? As we age, a number of connections between our hands and the parts of the brain that control them gradually decrease. As those connections diminish, so does the coordination between the brain and the hands. The signals and messages that the brain sends to the hands and fingers decrease. But the good news is that we can strengthen those signals by doing simple hand and finger exercises.

The following simple sets of special exercises will help increase:

- *Coordination of hand movements.*
- *Flexibility of the small joints in the hands and fingers.*
- *Blood circulation in the hands.*
- *Attention, ability to focus, and concentration.*

Exercise 4.1. Energize the Fingers

Step 1. Rub your palms together for several seconds. Move your hands slightly apart and then press your palms against each other (photo 4.1.1).

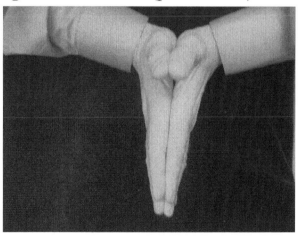

PHOTO **4.1.1**

Move your palms slightly apart, but keep the tips of your fingers pushed against each other (photo 4.1.2).

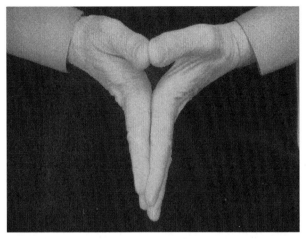

PHOTO 4.1.2

Step 2. Visualize that you are holding an imaginary ball between your palms (photo 4.1.3) and then press your fingers against each other.

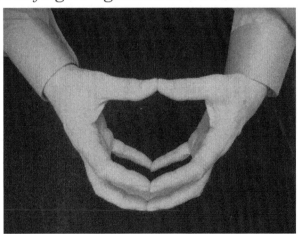

PHOTO 4.1.3

Then return back to holding your imaginary ball. Move your fingers close together (photo 4.1.4) and then back to the imaginary ball.

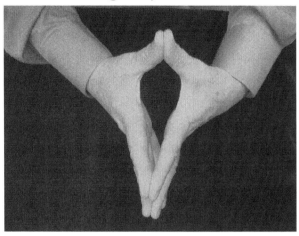

PHOTO 4.1.4

Begin to press all of your fingers together, as if you are pushing the air out of the ball (photo 4.1.5) and then return to the imaginary ball.

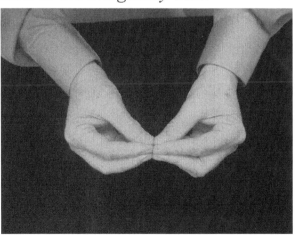

PHOTO 4.1.5

Step 3. Hold the tips of your thumbs and your index fingertips together (photo 4.1.6) and move them closer together (photo 4.1.7).

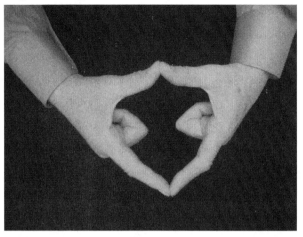

PHOTO 4.1.6

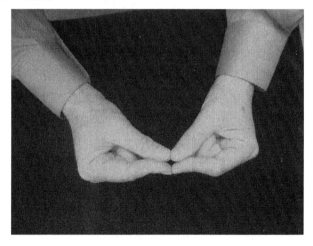

PHOTO 4.1.7

Repeat the same movements with your thumbs and your middle fingers (photo 4.1.8 and 4.1.9), with your thumbs and ring fingers and with your thumbs and pinkie fingers.

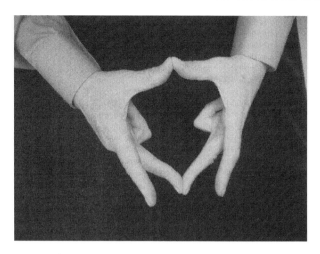

PHOTO **4.1.8**

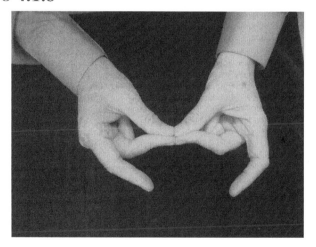

PHOTO **4.1.9**

Every movement has to be repeated from five to ten times.

Exercise 4.2. Energize the Fingers (continued)

Keep your fingers together, with your palms apart, facing up. Touch the sides of your hands against each other (photo 4.2.1) and bring your palms apart again.

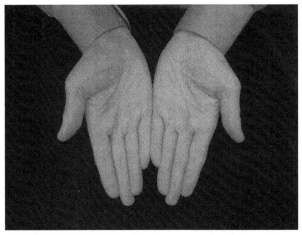

PHOTO 4.2.1

Now, touch the spaces between your thumbs and index fingers together (photo 4.2.2) and bring your palms apart again.

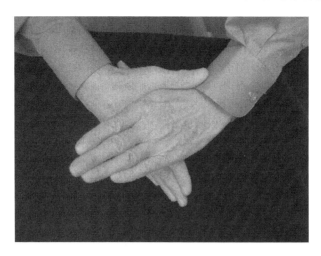

PHOTO **4.2.2**
Then, interlock your fingers (photo 4.2.3), and then move them apart.

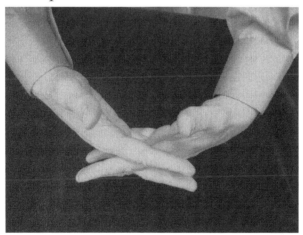

PHOTO **4.2.3**
Next, bring your fingers together and rub your thumbs together in a circular massaging motion for fifteen to thirty seconds (photo 4.2.4).

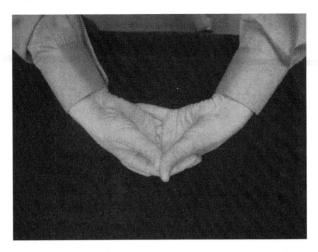

PHOTO **4.2.4**

Every element of these exercises has to be repeated five to ten times.

Exercise 4.3. Spirals in Space

Bring your palms together and use them to "draw" imaginary spirals in the air. Bend your arms at the elbows. Inhale and exhale as you bring your palms together in front of your chest.

Over the next three breathing cycles, say the sound "OM" as you exhale. Focus your attention on your fingertips. Make sure your eyes closely monitor the movements of your fingers. At the end of the exercises, say the sound "OM" three times again. Repeat these exercises three to five times.

4.3.1. *Begin "drawing" a spiral moving clockwise, gradually widening the size (width or radius) of the spiral (Figure 9).*

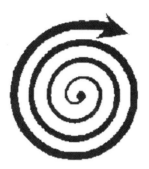

FIGURE 9.

Repeat the movement in the opposite direction, moving counterclockwise, and gradually narrow the size or radius of the spiral (Figure 10).

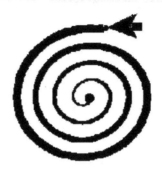

FIGURE 10.
Rest for fifteen to thirty seconds, breathing calmly.

4.3.2. Repeat the exercise. This time, begin "drawing" the spiral counterclockwise, widening the radius. Then, "draw" the spiral clockwise, narrowing the radius. Rest for fifteen to thirty seconds, breathing calmly.

4.3.3. With your palms pressed together, "draw" a double spiral (Figure 11), moving clockwise.

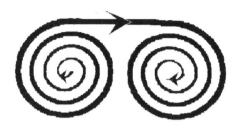

FIGURE **11.**
Start with a left spiral, and then move to the right spiral. Repeat the movement in the opposite direction, moving counterclockwise. Start with the right spiral, and then move to the left spiral. Rest for fifteen to thirty seconds, breathing calmly.

Exercise 4.4. Figure 8 and Petals

In this exercise, you will bring your palms together and use them to "draw" an imaginary figure 8 and petals in the air.

Bend your arms at the elbows. Inhale and exhale as you bring your palms together in front of your chest. Over the next three breathing cycles, say the sound "OM" as you exhale.

Focus your attention on your fingertips. Make sure your eyes closely monitor the movements of your fingers. At the end of the exercises, say the sound "OM" three times again.

4.4.1. Draw the Figure 8 in Space
Step 1. Begin moving your hands up and to the right, then down and to the left, "drawing" a small figure 8. Continue to draw larger and larger figure 8s. Then draw smaller and smaller figure 8s, until you reach the size of your original figure 8. (Figure 12).

Numbers

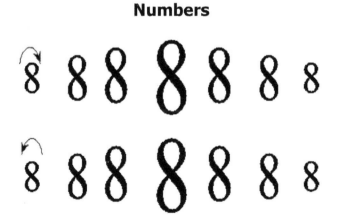

FIGURE 12.
Rest for fifteen to thirty seconds, breathing calmly.

Step 2. Repeat the exercise, moving up and to the left, then up and to the right. Rest for fifteen to thirty seconds, breathing calmly.

4.4.2. Draw Petals in Space

Step 1. Begin moving your hands up and to the right, then down and to the left, "drawing" a small flower petal. Draw larger and larger petals. Then draw smaller and smaller petals, until you reach the size of your original petal (Figure 13).

Petals

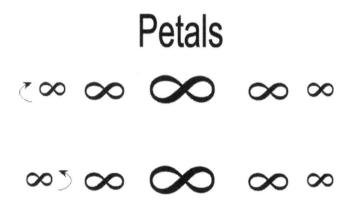

FIGURE 13.
Rest for fifteen to thirty seconds, breathing calmly.

Step 2. Repeat the exercise in opposite direction, moving hands up and to the left, then up and to the

Valentin Bragin, M.D.

right. Rest for fifteen to thirty seconds, breathing calmly.

Exercise 4.5. Numbers in Space

Holding your palms together, "draw" imaginary numbers in the air. (Figure 14).

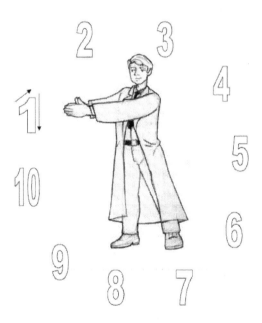

FIGURE 14.

Inhale and "draw" the number 1, as you exhale. Repeat the exercise, drawing higher and higher numbers, until you reach the number 10.

Exercise 4.6. Geometric Figures in Space

Holding your palms together, "draw" imaginary geometric figures in the air.

Draw ten triangles.
Draw ten squares.
Draw ten circles.

Exercise 4.7. Stretching Exercise—the Ring

These exercises require that you use your imagination. Holding your fingertips tightly together, imagine that a rubber band is holding them together. As you move your fingers apart, imagine how the rubber band will stretch.

Step 1. First step, the exercise should be performed simultaneously with both hands.

Inhale and bring your thumbs to your index fingers. Picture the rubber band stretched around your fingers (photo 4.7.1).

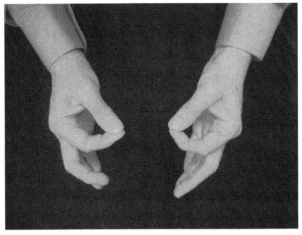

PHOTO 4.7.1.

Exhale. As you exhale, stretch the imaginary rubber band, moving your fingers as far apart as you can (photo 4.7.2).

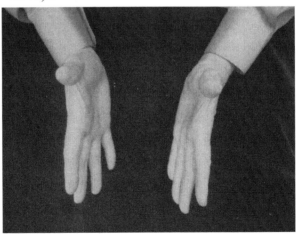

PHOTO 4.7.2.

Repeat the same exercise using your thumb and middle finger, (photo 4.7.3), then your thumb and ring finger, and finally, your thumb and pinkie finger.

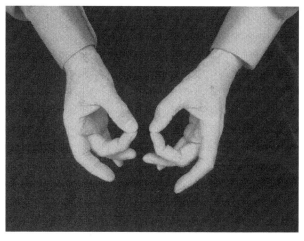

PHOTO **4.7.3.**

Step 2. Repeat the exercise using each hand separately.

Exercise 4.8. The Pencil

You will rotate a pencil between your fingers.

Step 1. With your palms facing down, tighten both hands around a pencil. Begin rotating the pencil horizontally with both hands (photo 4.8.1).

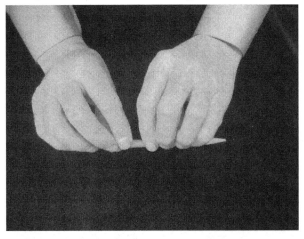

PHOTO 4.8.1.

Without pausing, gradually lift each finger, so that you rotate the pencil with fewer and fewer fingers (photos 4.8.2, 4.8.3).

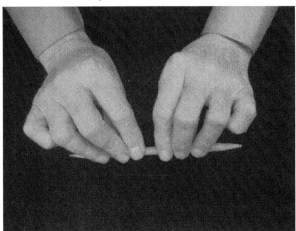

PHOTO 4.8.2

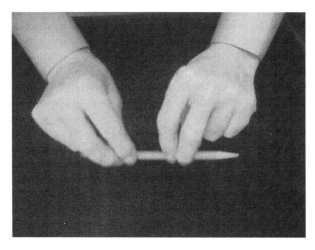

PHOTO **4.8.3.**

Then, rotate the pencil with only your index and ring fingers (photo 4.8.4) and with your index and pinkie fingers.

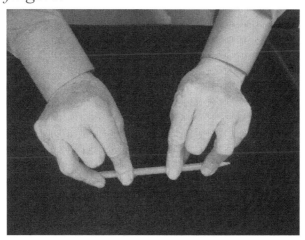

PHOTO **4.8.4.**

Valentin Bragin, M.D.

Step 2. Place the pencil vertically in your right hand and begin rotating it (photo 4.8.5).

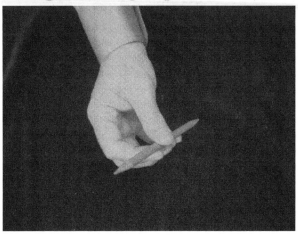

PHOTO 4.8.5.

Without pausing, gradually lift each finger, starting with pinkie finger. Continue pencil rotation vertically with your thumb, index, and ring fingers (photo 4.8.6).

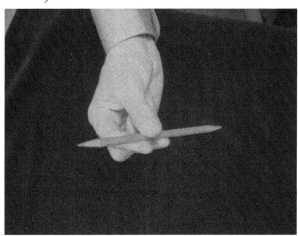

PHOTO 4.8.6.

Without pausing, use your thumb, middle, and pinkie fingers, and finally with the thumb, index, and pinkie fingers (photo 4.8.7).

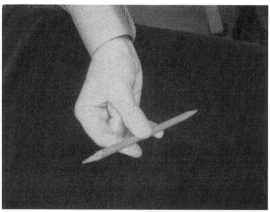

PHOTO **4.8.7.**

Step 3. Repeat the exercise using your left hand.
Step 4. Repeat Step 1.

Exercise 4.9. The Tennis Ball

You will touch a tennis ball with your fingers and release your fingers. Focus all your attention on the moment your fingers touch the ball. You do not need to squeeze the ball or exert any pressure on it; just loosely touch it. As you do the exercise, breathe evenly, but not too deeply. Do not hold your breath.

Step 1. Begin rotating the ball between your palms (photo 4.9.1).

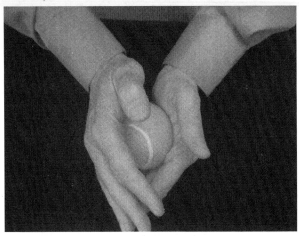

PHOTO 4.9.1.

Try to touch the ball with the entire surface of your palms.

Step 2. Now, take the ball in your right hand and knock it lightly against the palm of your left hand five or six times (photo 4.9.2).

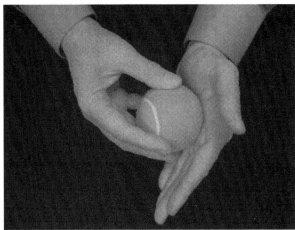

PHOTO 4.9.2.

Switch hands and repeat the exercise (photo 4.9.3).

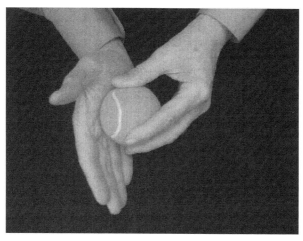

PHOTO 4.9.3.

Step 3. Place the ball between your palms. Cup your hands in a V shape (photo 4.9.4).

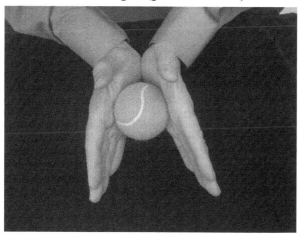

PHOTO 4.9.4.

Touch the ball with the fingers of your right hand (photo 4.9.5) and then left hand (photo 4.9.6) by alternating your hands. As you continue, repeat this motion.

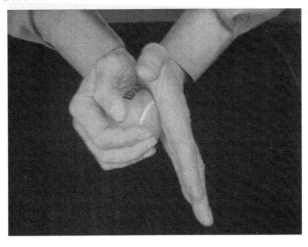

PHOTO **4.9.5.**

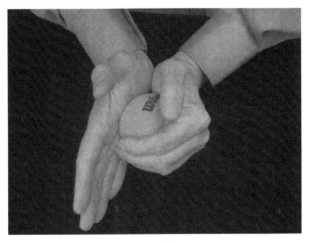

PHOTO **4.9.6**

Step 4. Place your palms parallel to each other (photo 4.9.7).

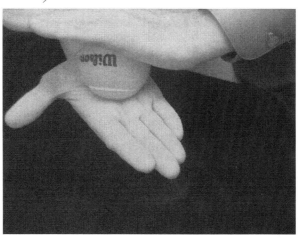

PHOTO 4.9.7.

Hold the ball between your palms. Imagine that you are making a snowball. Touch the ball with the fingers of both hands, and then straighten your fingers (photo 4.9.8).

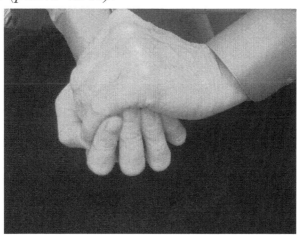

PHOTO 4.9.8.

Step 5. Repeat Step 2.

The length of each of the steps in this exercise is one to two minutes, for a total exercise time of five to ten minutes.

Exercise 4.10. Stretching Exercise—the Lock

You can use this simple exercise to alleviate drowsiness, which people sometimes experience after performing meditation or breathing exercises.

Interlock the fingers of both hands, with your palms facing you.

Then, turn your locked hands with the palms facing away from you. Stretch your forearms carefully until you feel slight tension in the fingers and palms of both hands. Hold your arms in this position for five to ten seconds. Now, bend your arms at the elbows slowly and turn your locked hands back so that the palms are again facing you as they were at the start of the exercise.

5. Legs

As we grow older, our gait changes; we walk slower and lose steadiness and smoothness. Foot exercises activate zones within the cerebral cortex, the part of the brain that represents legs, improving blood circulation in the legs and flexibility of foot joints, and strengthening the arches of the feet.

Exercise 5.1. The Warm-Up

Sit in a comfortable position with your feet flat on the floor.

Curl and uncurl your toes.

Slightly lift your toes and turn both your feet simultaneously to the right, then to the left. Then slightly lift your toes and turn your right foot to the right, while at the same time, turning your left foot to the left.

The toes on both your feet will go up and down, and both will be moving at the same time. Then, as the toes on the right foot go up, the toes on the left foot go down, alternating in this way.

Exercise 5.2. High Heels

This exercise is very beneficial for people who spend a lot of time in a sitting position. It helps with blood circulation in the legs.

In the first part of the exercise, your heels will go up and down at different speeds.

In the second part of the exercise, you will be asked to concentrate on the warm sensation in your legs created by these movements.

Each cycle consists of ten repetitive movements, approximately one half inch from the floor. The first three movements are slower (one movement per second), and then the next seven movements are faster (two movements per second).

While doing exercises, pay attention to the feelings and sensations in the feet. Any unpleasant sensation in your legs is a sign that you should stop the exercise. Do not push yourself to exhaustion.

Part 1.

Sit in a comfortable position with your feet on the floor. Close your eyes and place all your concentration on your feet.

Start the first cycle by counting one number per second in your head 1 - 2 - 3, then count faster (two numbers per second) 4-5 - 6-7 - 8-9 - 10.

Each time you complete an exercise by counting up to ten, it is one set of the exercise. Now continue, but this time do two sets of the exercise. Finally, repeat the exercise, but do three sets. Then, stop all movements and observe your reaction. Repeat this exercise one to two times a day. Gradually increase the frequency of the exercises, up to four or five sets a day. When you feel comfortable, continue to increase the number of sets to ten (one hundred movements total).

Part 2.

After you complete Part 1 of the exercise, you will probably have warm feelings in your feet and ankles. To strengthen the sensation, you can use a visualization or imagination technique. Here's how it works:

> *Picture yourself in your mind on the beach. Imagine it in your mind as vividly as possible.*
>
> *Close your eyes.*
>
> *Take several breaths.*
>
> *Focus your attention on your feet.*
>
> *Imagine that you are on the beach.*
>
> *It's a bright, sunny day.*
>
> *The sand is pleasantly hot.*
>
> *You are standing on the sand.*
>
> *Feel the pleasant warmth that radiates into your feet from the sand.*
>
> *The warmth rises higher and higher, spreading to your shins and reaching your thighs.*
>
> *You feel the pleasant sensations, warmth, and relaxation all throughout your legs.*
>
> *You experience pleasant sensations, warmth, and relaxation.*
>
> *The warm feeling is getting stronger. Remember this sensation.*
>
> *Take several breaths and then open your eyes.*

Notice how long it takes for this sensation to disappear.

6. The Spine

It is well known that our health and longevity depend on the flexibility of the spine and the strength of the muscles that support the spine. As we get older, the spine becomes stiffer and more rigid.

The neck area is especially important for brain functions. This area contains arteries that feed blood into the back portion of the brain, including the cerebellum, which is responsible for body balance. Any problems in the neck (muscle spasms, vertebral misalignment, muscle atrophy, bad posture) could easily interrupt the blood supply to the brain and cause headaches, vision problems, neck and shoulder pain, numbness in the hands, dizzy spells, gait changes, and many other problems.

Additionally, there are also many nervous system pathways between the neck and the brain. To illustrate the importance of neck-brain connections, think of the way a cat carries her kitten, grabbing the kitten by the back of the neck, which immediately causes the kitten to lose balance and leg coordination.

The aim of the following exercises is to fortify the muscles in the neck, shoulders, and chest areas; to increase flexibility of the spine in the neck area; and to improve the mobility of the shoulders.

Do these exercises in a seated position with full attention on the neck and shoulder areas. The head is in an upright position and your eyes are looking straight ahead. Try not to move your head while doing these exercises. Each cycle consists of ten movements that will be repeated in clockwise and counterclockwise directions. In the beginning, you will do two or three of these cycles of exercises before stopping. Gradually increase the number of cycles to ten (for a total of one hundred movements).

Exercise 6.1. Rotate Your Shoulders

Shrug your shoulders up and then rotate them back, down, forward, and up again. Repeat these rotations in the opposite direction (Figure 15).

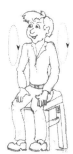

FIGURE **15**

Exercise 6.2. Shrug Your Shoulders Up and Down

Shrug your shoulders up and then back down. Inhale while you are doing the up movement and exhale while you are doing the down movement (Figure 16).

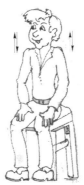

FIGURE 16

Exercise 6.3. Rotate Your Arms around Your Torso and Head

6.3.1. Rest both of your hands on your thighs. Do not change the position of your head. Your concentration is on the process of your hands' movements. Start this exercise with your right arm resting on your right thigh. Begin moving your right arm. Bring your right arm up in front of the torso toward the left side, bypass the left ear, back of the head, right ear and bring it back down to your right thigh. Without touching your right knee, start the same movement again and repeat five to ten times.

6.3.2. Repeat exercise 6.3.1, moving your right hand in the opposite direction. Bring your right arm up in front of the torso toward the right ear. Then bypass the back of the head and the left ear and bring it back down to your right thigh. Repeat the same movements five to ten times.

6.3.3. Repeat exercise 6.3.1 using your left hand.

6.3.4. Repeat exercise 6.3.2 using your left hand.

7. Combination Exercises

Combination exercises activate the brain through several sensory channels at the same time. This exercise activates the sensory-motor zones of the brain's cortex that corresponds to the arms and legs.

Exercise 7.1. "The Rhythm"

Place your hands on your knees, palms facing down. Put your feet firmly on the floor. Exercises 7.1.1. through 7.1.3 are based on the simultaneous movements of hands and feet in the same directions. Each exercise consists of five to ten movements.

7.1.1. Fingers of your right hand and toes of your right foot or fingers of your left hand and toes of your left foot.

Move the fingers of your right hand up and down, while keeping your feet still.
Move the toes of your right foot up and down, while keeping your hands still.
Move both your right fingers and right toes up and down.
Repeat these same sequences of the movements using fingers of your left hand and toes of your left foot.

7.1.2. Fingers of your right and left hands or toes of your right and left feet.

Move both your right and left fingers, while keeping your feet still.

Move both your right and left toes, while keeping your fingers still.
Move both your right and left fingers and toes up and down.

7.1.3. Fingers of your right hand and toes of your left foot or fingers of your left hand and toes of your right foot.

Move the fingers of your right hand and toes of your left foot up and down.
Move the fingers of your left hand and toes of your right foot up and down.

Part III:
Memory Training Exercises

There are many useful techniques and books that describe different memory training exercises.[7, 8, 9, 10, 16, 17, 18] But most of those books are dedicated to healthy people. There are not too many sources that specifically address the needs of elderly and disabled people.

But elderly and disabled people still have some of their brain reserves left, which can be used for memory training. The following exercises are some examples of concentration and memory training, which we have implemented for our patients.

These exercises are based on the fact that information flows into the brain through multi-channel sensory systems and is then stored in different parts of the brain.

In other words, information we take in through hearing, seeing, listening, reading, or other sources goes to the brain through various channels, and then the brain stores it in its own system of file cabinets—or the different sections of the brain.

Recently, different locations in the brain were discovered for storing and processing information such as words, numbers, objects, faces, shapes, and colors. This data gives us an opportunity to work with these certain areas of the brain, while doing memory training. For successful concentration and memory training, the person has to do multiple repetitions of the training exercises.

These exercises are even more effective—and fun—if you do them with a friend who can help you keep track of the results. At the end of each exercise, spend five minutes doing breathing exercises and then try to recall the information you've memorized.

8. Examples of Memory Training Exercises

Exercise 8.1. Memorizing Objects

8.1.1. Objects. There are pictures of different objects (Figure 17).

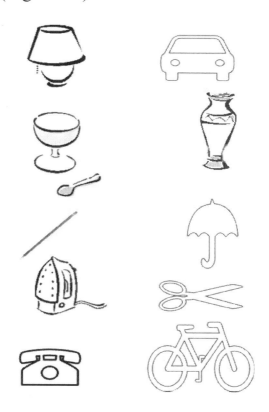

FIGURE 17

*Study these objects for several seconds and try
to memorize them.*

*Close the book. Try to recall the objects shown
in the pictures.*

*Open the book and check your results to see how
many objects you remembered.*

*Repeat this exercise ten times, or until you can
remember all the objects on the page.*

Spend five minutes doing breathing exercises.
After you've completed the breathing exercises, try
to recall the objects again.

8.1.2. Individual Cards with Objects

For this exercise, you will need to find various
cards with objects on them. Begin with five to seven
different cards, and then gradually increase the
number of cards.

*Place the cards on the table. Study them for
several seconds. Try to memorize the details
of the cards. Then place a sheet of blank paper
over the cards.*

*Try to recall as many cards as you can. Write
them down.*

Remove the paper and check your results.

Repeat this exercise ten times, or until you can remember the maximum number of cards on the table.

Rest five minutes, then try to recall the cards again.

The next time you do this exercise, select a different set of cards.

8.1.3. Real Objects

For this exercise, you will need to select real objects such as pens, small toys, multicolored bits of cloth, keys of various shapes, pencils, coins, postcards, etc.

As an example, let's use pens or pencils that are different colors.

Place the objects on the table. Study them. Pick them up, if necessary.
Place a blank sheet of paper over the objects.
Try to recall the objects, their color, and their positions on the table.
Write them down.
Remove the paper and check your results.
Repeat this exercise ten times, or until you can remember all the objects on the table.

Rest five minutes, then try to recall the objects again.

The next time you do this exercise, select a different set of objects.

Exercise 8.2. Memorizing Pictures with Numbers

On the following pages are pictures of various objects with numbers associated with them (Figure 18).

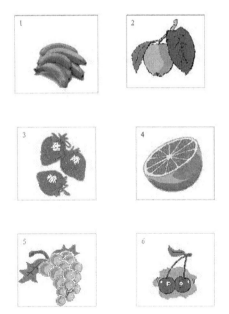

FIGURE 18

Study the page for several seconds.

Try to memorize the pictures and their numbers.

Close the book.

Try to recall the objects shown in the pictures and their numbers.

Open the book and check your results.

Repeat this exercise ten times, or until you can remember all the pictures on the page and their numbers.

Spend five minutes doing breathing exercises. After you've completed the breathing exercises, try to recall the pictures and their numbers again.

Exercise 8.3. Memorizing Geometric Shapes

The following pages show various geometric shapes (Figure 19).

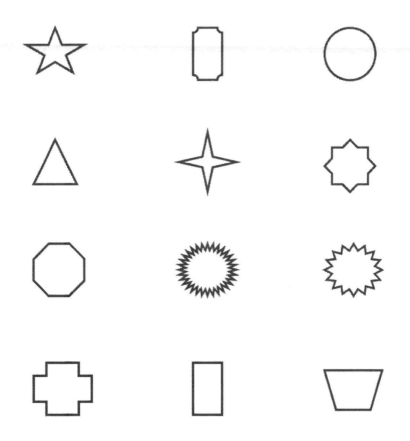

FIGURE 19

Study the page for several seconds.

Try to memorize the geometric shapes.

Close the book.

Try recalling the shapes in the pictures.

Open the book and check your results.

Repeat this exercise ten times, or until you can remember all the geometric shapes on the page.

Spend five minutes doing breathing exercises. After you've completed the breathing exercises, try to recall the geometric shapes again.

Part IV:
Other Ways to Activate the Brain

Actually, almost any kind of routine you can think of can be useful for working with the brain to stimulate and activate it. All you have to do is gently focus your attention on whatever activity you happen to be doing at the time, and you will already be on the way to activating your brain in a healthy way.

Nutrition, sound, music, and light all help to naturally activate the brain. Many books have been written on the subject. In this section of the workbook, there is only brief coverage of these topics. People can easily and naturally activate their brains through these simple techniques.

9. Nutrition

Nutrition has a powerful effect on the brain's functions. Food activates the brain in many different ways. For example, the brain can be stimulated by seeing food, smelling it, and of course by touching and tasting it.

We have all experienced how just thinking about our favorite food can trigger a reaction in our brain. If we see or smell food—or even hear it sizzle as it cooks—the brain automatically triggers the digestive system and prepares the body for eating.

When we put food in our mouths, the teeth chew it, the tongue tastes it, and the brain becomes even more involved. As we chew our food, the brain sends signals to organize the digestive process. The body begins to release enzymes and other chemicals, based on the type of food we are eating. When we digest our food nicely, the brain also signals feelings of satisfaction, so that we don't feel hungry but rather feel full.

The brain can even remember every kind of food we've ever tasted or eaten. For example, if we eat the same breakfast every morning, our brain memorizes the menu and triggers the release of digestive juices for those particular kinds of foods. This special memory helps the brain control the production of those chemicals and enzymes that give us the best digestion based on the foods we eat.

The brain can easily recall meals we ate as children. This memory might cause mixed emotions. The meals we love always give us warm and pleasant memories, and that is our "comfort food." But the foods we were forced to eat against our will can cause unpleasant thoughts and emotions.

Here is a simple yet powerful example. In childhood, for some people, taking a spoonful of cod liver oil was a very unpleasant experience. Decades later, many of these people still refuse to take any kind of fish oil, even when they are fully aware that it is a healthy tonic for the heart and the brain.

The brain makes sure the organs of the digestive tract are working together properly. The way we absorb food and nutrition changes, depending on brain activity, and what the body may need for energy and growth. That is why people lose their appetite when they feel depressed or upset. The brain activity affects our digestion.

Let's talk a little bit about how the digestive system and the different organs of the body break down the food we eat. As you know, the food we see on our plate contains vitamins, minerals, fats, carbohydrates, and proteins. The food is transformed by digestive system enzymes into amino acids, peptides (several amino acids, binding together) fatty acids, and simple carbohydrates (glucose, fructose), which are absorbed into the walls of the intestines and reach the liver. In the liver, there are assembly lines for the synthesis of different body proteins, fats, and carbohydrates. A certain amount of amino acids, free fatty acids, and glucose are going directly into the bloodstream and then to the different organs and tissues.

Every organ uses food for an energy supply and for the synthesis of organ-specific proteins like muscle proteins, receptors, membranes, and so on. For an energy supply, the body cells need glucose, fructose, free fatty acids, and in certain conditions, amino acids. The heart is not very picky—it can consume any nutritional element from the blood (amino acids, glucose, ketone bodies, and fatty acids). The brain utilizes only glucose and ketone bodies to work. The muscles also need glucose, but can use fatty acids as well. For synthesis, the cells need mostly amino acids, especially essential amino acids, and a relatively small amount of glucose and free fatty acids. During stress, the synthesis processes in the body temporary slow down, and the main flow of nutrients switches over to energy supply to meet extra demands on our organs.

There are no special foods required to replenish energy. We get energy from proteins, carbohydrates, and fat, which are found in all kinds of food. But to build or to repair the body, food has to contain special and important types of nutrients, which the body cannot produce on its own. These include vitamins, essential amino acids, fatty acids, and microelements.

Vitamins are essential for the brain to function in a healthy, active way. For example, if we don't get enough only of one vitamin—Vitamin B1—it may cause problems of the heart, alter our brain activity, and lead to depression. Popular opinion says that we get enough vitamins with our food, but unfortunately, this is not always the case.

It is a well-known fact that people of advanced age often suffer from poor digestion, irregularity, and a lack of absorption of vitamins into the bloodstream. I often find that my patients have low levels of vitamin B12. A lack of sufficient vitamin B12 is connected to memory problems, difficulty with walking and balance, and anemia.

Supplements play an important role in maintaining vital body functions. Some supplements improve the functions of certain organs; others help produce energy and regenerate or repair cells in the body. Our brain activity and psychological state—or state of mind—have a great influence on digestion. Stress interrupts healthy digestion in every part of the gastrointestinal system.

While eating, you should avoid talking about any topics that might cause anxiety and bad thoughts. Before you begin your meal, take time to relax, take a few deep breaths, observe the food in front of you, and then begin eating in a stress-free, relaxed state of mind.

Water is absolutely necessary for normal brain and body functions. For example, water can sometimes quickly cure fatigue. But as we grow older, many of us lose the feeling of thirst. It can lead to dehydration and disruption of our brain functions. When that happens, we may feel upset or agitated, and confused or disoriented. We recommend that you drink between a quart and a quart and a half of water each day. Start your day with a drink of one or one and a half glasses of water, thirty minutes before breakfast. This water must be fresh, not carbonated, and without juice, sugar, or lemon. The water will be quickly absorbed and will have an uplifting effect on the body.

Things added to water (such as carbonation, honey, juice, lemon, or sugar) turn water into food, as far as the brain is concerned. The brain believes that this "water" is food, and triggers the digestive enzymes' cascade. For that reason, it is important to drink fresh, plain water daily, in addition to whatever other food or drinks you might enjoy.

Now, let's talk about diet. Diet is a word that turns many people off or frightens them. Who needs dieting? Our favorite kind of diet is a "see-food" diet. We just eat whatever we see! But "diet" should not be seen as a "four-letter word." Let me assure you that your diet is as important for your health as drinking water, doing exercises, or taking vitamins and medications. I have to tell my patients over and over that their treatment starts with the food on their plate. We all know that people suffering from joint diseases, heart conditions, diabetes, and many other ailments benefit from following a certain kind of diet. A healthy and balanced diet can save your life and keep you active for years to come.

When you consider following a diet, you must consciously select the food products that have a positive and healing effect on your body. At the same time, you must limit the foods which affect your health negatively. Diet triggers many significant changes in brain and body functions, as well as changes in our metabolism.

My recommendations for diet are very simple: Start with one healthy meal a day, and then pay attention to how it makes you feel. Compare it to the rest of your meals. Then slowly change the second meal to a "diet" meal. Gradually, you will begin to feel different and better. Your mind will become sharper and your body will have more energy.

Bookstores are full of books describing diets of every sort. Which diet is better? The answer is that the best diet for you is the one that makes you feel comfortable and helps you lead a normal, healthy life. Food is your weapon to improve your health and to fight against disease.

10. Sounds and Music

Sound plays a special role in brain development and activity. The brain begins to respond to different sounds and rhythms when a child is still in the womb. After birth, sound surrounds the baby, and the baby learns to make sounds of his or her own. Eventually, the moment comes when the child begins to use sounds to express feelings and to talk.

Before the child's brain can figure out what words actually mean, it first reacts to the tone, volume, and pitch of other people's voices. Certain sounds can relax muscles, relieve tension, and sharpen attention. As an example, you can be soothed by the sound of rain, the ocean, or singing birds. Other sounds can cause stress and muscle tension, and hamper the functioning of the brain. Loud sounds can even cause ear damage, shock, and trauma.

The brain's reaction to certain sounds and musical pieces depends on its previous exposure to them. The rush of falling water or the whisper of the ocean might not sound pleasant to some people, while others find these sounds so relaxing that they might even doze off while listening to them.

Music can have calming or stimulating effects on the brain. To obtain a calming effect, listen to Chopin's *Nocturnes.* To experience a stimulating effect, listen to Ravel's *Bolero,* fast drumming, or marching band music. Classical music (like Vivaldi, Bach, and Beethoven) has the ability to both calm and stimulate the brain at the same time, depending on our state of mind as well as the particular piece of music we select.

Songs and melodies of our youth have a great effect on brain activity, no matter how old we are. They trigger memories of times past and carry corresponding emotional reactions. Many of these songs cause strong positive emotions. I strongly recommend singing songs that you remember, and which evoke warm, comforting feelings.

11. Exposure to Light

Light acts as a natural stimulus for our nervous system. Natural daylight helps our "body clock" to function and release the hormones or chemicals in the brain that are responsible for helping us fall asleep and get a good night's rest. The natural light we get during the day also helps us to wake up and be alert the next morning.

Low-level or dim light changes brain activity right away. For example, what is going on in the brain of a person who is alone in a forest without a flashlight when the sun goes down? The brain becomes more active and alert, and tries to get more information about the surroundings. This person stops walking, looks around carefully, and listens for even the smallest sound. The pupils dilate, the hearing becomes more sensitive, and one moves more slowly through the forest.

A decrease in indoor light has the same kind of effect on people of advanced age. As we become older, our reaction to darkness changes because of vision and hearing problems. People feel tired, withdrawn, irritable, depressed, and anxious. Some elderly people even experience agitation or become drowsy because of changes related to a lack of light. People feel half-asleep in the daytime and then have trouble sleeping at night.

I often see people spend the whole day indoors in a semi-dark room, with the curtains closed. Light is barely reaching them. Many of them become angry or disturbed when the curtains are opened. A recent study showed that "daylight lamps"—special lamps that give off light spectrums that are similar to real sunlight—have a positive effect on elderly people in nursing homes. People have more contacts with each other, experience less fatigue, and improve balance and walking.

Since the beginning of time, people have used various colors to stimulate or relax the nervous system. Red and yellow shades—that can be found in bright, colorful paintings or photographs filled with red or yellow colors—stimulate and excite the brain. Green and blue hues calm the brain, and help to lower anxiety and relieve worry. We often see these colors in paintings of the sea or in relaxing landscapes. Studies even show that the color blue can help to alleviate pain.

Concluding Remarks

You are about to finish reading this book and turn the last page. I hope that you received helpful, useful, and valuable information about brain activation exercises.

In the coming years, we will all bear witness to new research and insight into the brain and its functions. Unfortunately, the practical application of that kind of research could be many years away. This program, however, is practical and easy to implement right now. Even those patients who have serious medical conditions can use it.

You can easily create and design your own individual brain activation program, by choosing one exercise from each part of the book. You can use this set of exercises for several weeks and then switch to another one. Along the way, you will learn how the brain and body work together—and find new ways to activate the brain's functions to make your body more healthy and energetic.

I wish you good health for many years to come.

Valentin Bragin, M.D.

Selected References

1. Kabat-Zinn, J. *Full Catastrophe Living: Using the Wisdom of Your Body and Mind to Face Stress, Pain, and Illness.* New York: Delta, 1991.
2. Bragin, V. *How to Activate Your Brain.* New York: Mir Collection, 2005, in Russian.
3. Wallace, W. C., V. Bragin, N.K. Robakis, K. Sambamurti, D. VanderPutten, C.R. Merril, K.L. Davis, A.C. Santucci, and V. Haroutunian. "Increased biosynthesis of Alzheimer amyloid precursor protein in the cerebral cortex of rats with lesions of the nucleus basalis of Meynert." *Molecular Brain Research,* 10:173-178 (1991).
4. Wallace, W., S.T. Ahlers, J. Gotlib, V. Bragin, J. Sugar, R. Gluck, P.A. Shea, K.L. Davis, and V. Haroutunian. "Amyloid precursor protein in the cerebral cortex is rapidly and persistently induced by loss of subcortical innervation." *Proc. Natl. Acad. Sci. U.S.A.,* 90(18):8712-6 (1993).
5. Khalsa, G.S., and C. Stauth. *Brain Longevity.* New York: Warner Books, 1997.
6. Bragin, V., M. Chemodanova, I. Bragin, J. Polyak, and I. Slepchina. "Monitoring Autonomic Nervous System Response

after Sensory-Motor Stimulation Exercises by Using Heart Rate Variability." Poster presented at the Conference on Prevention of Dementia: Early Diagnosis and Intervention; July 18-21, Washington, D.C., S60, (2005).

7. Fotuhi, M. *The Memory Cure*, New York: McGraw-Hill, 2003.

8. Katz, L.C., and M. Rubin. *Keep Your Brain Alive.* New York: Workman Publishing Company, 1999.

9. Small, G. *The Memory Bible.* New York: Hyperion, 2002.

10. Wetzel, K., and K. Harmeyer. *Mind Games.* Albany, New York: Delmar Thomson Learning, 2000.

11. Ivanov I.I., U.U. Keerig, V.I. Bragin, A.I. Zaytsev, V.A. Shindin, L.I. Haykina, and V.K. Nebishinetz. "Changes in fraction composition in various types of rabbit's muscles in onthogenesis." *Journal of Evolutional Biochemistry and Physiology.* 3:717-719 (1967), in Russian.

12. Goldberg, E. *The Wisdom Paradox: How Your Mind Can Grow Stronger as Your Brain Grows Older.* New York: Gotham, 2005.

13. Schwartz, J.M., and S. Begley. *The Mind and the Brain.* New York: HarperCollins, 2002.

14. Lu, B. "BDNF and activity-dependent synaptic modulation." *Learn Mem.,* Mar-Apr; 10 (2):86-98 (2003).

15. Bragin, V., M. Chemodanova, N. Dzhafarova, I. Bragin, J.L. Czerniawski, and G. Aliev. "Integrated treatment approach improves cognitive function in demented and clinically depressed patients." *American Journal of Alzheimer's Disease and Other Dementias;* Jan.-Feb., 20(1):21-26 (2005).

16. Noir, M., and B. Croisile. *Dental Floss for the Mind.* New York: McGraw-Hill, 2005.

17. Perlmutter, D. *BrainRecovery.com.* Naples, Florida: The Perlmutter Health Center, 2000.

18. Stein D., S. Brailowsky, and B. Will. *Brain Repair.* New York: Oxford University Press, 1997.

Useful links

The Alzheimer's Association
http://www.alz.org

Alzheimer's Disease Education and Referral (ADEAR)
Center
http://www.alzheimers.org

The National Institute on Aging Information Center
http://www.nia.nih.gov

The Alzheimer's Foundation of America Reach Out for
Care
http://www.alzfdn.org

The American Geriatric Society
http://www.americangeriatrics.org

American Association of Retired Persons (AARP)
http://www.aarp.org

Integrative approach to the brain:
http://www.2020brainpower.com/

Nutrition:
http://www.healthrecipes.com

Information:
http://www.alzheimersdailynews.com
http://www.seniorjornal.com

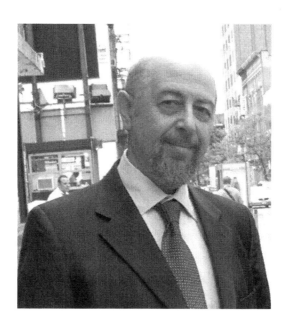

About the Author

Valentin Bragin, M.D., Ph.D., is a psychiatrist and the founder and medical director of the Stress Relief and Memory Training Center (SRMTC) in Brooklyn, New York, where more than 2,000 patients have been treated within the first 12 years of its operation.

Dr. Bragin graduated and earned his Ph.D. from one of the oldest and most prestigious medical schools in the former Soviet Union, the Russian Medical Military Academy in Leningrad. Dr. Bragin also holds an engineering degree in computer science (medical informatics).

His areas of interest include stress and stress-related disorders, aging, and rehabilitation of brain functions in people with cognitive problems. He has dedicated many years of his medical career to researching the impact of stress on illness and overall health.

For the last seven years, Dr. Bragin has focused on the preservation of cognitive functions in the elderly who suffer from memory loss and depression. His strategy involves an integrative treatment approach utilizing the brain's own reserves and resources, which can be activated at any age.

The foundation of his Brain Activation Program is a set of unique sensory-motor exercises that are presented in this book. Dr. Bragin enjoys using these exercises himself and strongly believes that they can slow down or at least postpone the process of memory decline. He continues to develop new and unique sensory-motor exercises.

The results of Dr. Bragin's treatment program have been presented at national and international conferences and have been published in the *American Journal of Alzheimer's Disease and Other Dementias* in 2005.

Dr. Bragin is the author of numerous publications.

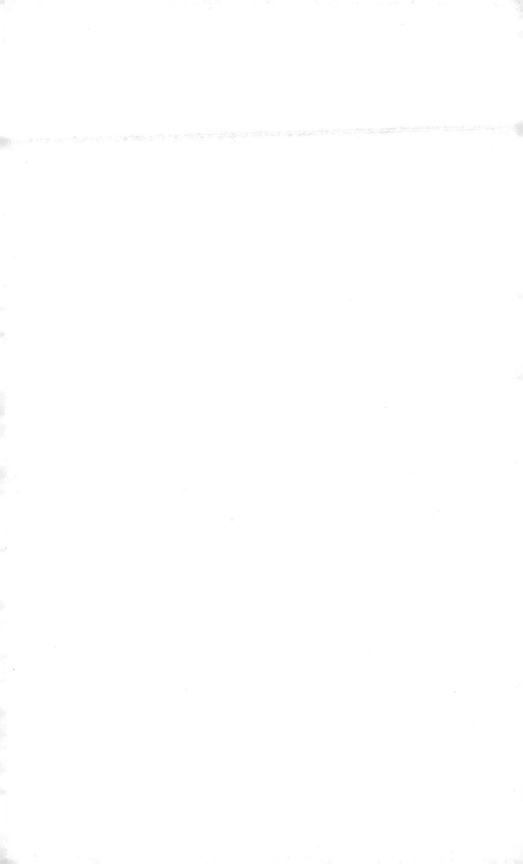

32055113R00100

Made in the USA
Middletown, DE
20 May 2016